MILAD

D0705785

STANDARD BARBERING
EXAM REVIEW

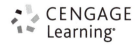

CENGAGE
Learning·

Australia • Brazil • Mexico • Singapore • United Kingdom • United States

CENGAGE
Learning·

Milady Standard Barbering Exam Review, 6th Edition

Executive Director, Milady: Sandra Bruce

Product Director: Corina Santoro

Content Developer: Sarah Prediletto

Associate Learning Design Author: Harry Garrott

Product Assistant: Michelle Whitehead

Senior Director, Sales & Marketing: Gerard McAvey

Marketing Manager: Elizabeth Bushey

Senior Director, Production: Wendy Troeger

Director, Production: Andrew Crouth

Senior Content Project Manager: Nina Tucciarelli

Senior Art Director: Benj Gleeksman

Cover Images:
  Hair: Fern Andong and Jes Sutton

  Makeup: Amy Elizabeth

  Photography: Joseph and Yuki Paradiso

Library of Congress Control Number: 2016934303

ISBN-13: 978-1-305-10067-1

Milady
20 Channel Center Street
Boston, MA 02210
USA

Cengage Learning is a leading provider of customized learning solutions with employees residing in nearly 40 different countries and sales in more than 125 countries around the world. Find your local representative at **www.cengage.com**.

Cengage Learning products are represented in Canada by Nelson Education, Ltd.

For your lifelong learning solutions, visit **milady.cengage.com**.

Purchase any of our products at your local college store or at our preferred online store **www.cengagebrain.com**.

Visit our corporate website at **cengage.com**.

Printed in the United States of America
Print Number: 05   Print Year: 2019

CONTENTS

PART *2* **SAMPLE STATE BOARD EXAMINATIONS**

PART *3* **ANSWER KEYS**

PREFACE

This book of exam reviews contains questions similar to those that may be found on state licensing exams for barbering. It employs multiple-choice questions, which have been widely adopted and approved by the majority of state licensing boards.

Groups of questions have been arranged following each chapter of the *Milady Standard Barbering* textbook. To get the maximum advantage when using this book, it is advisable that the review of subject matter take place shortly after its classroom presentation. After completing the chapter exams, use the answer key located in the back of the exam review to confirm the correct response. For this edition, the page number also appears, where you can locate the answer in *Milady Standard Barbering*.

This review book attempts to keep pace with and ensure a basic understanding of all topics needed to become a successful barber and complete your state board licensing exam.

While the exam review serves as an excellent guide for the student in preparing for their state licensing examination, it can also be beneficial for experienced barbers. It provides a reliable standard against which professionals can measure their knowledge, understanding, and abilities.

Furthermore, reviewing this material will help students and professionals alike to gain a more thorough understanding of the full scope of their work as they answer questions regarding practical performance skills and related theory. Because the practice tests are written for the most recent edition of the *Milady Standard Barbering* textbook, use of this material by professionals also helps to ensure that they have the most recent knowledge and information available to them in the industry.

1 THE HISTORY OF BARBERING

MULTIPLE CHOICE

1. Archaeological studies have shown that simple implements were made to cut hair using _____, _____, and _____.
   a. sharpened flints, oyster shells, bone
   b. twigs, rocks, vines
   c. steel, rubber, ivory
   d. stone, brass, shells   ____

2. Many primitive cultures had belief systems that elevated tribal barbers to positions of importance; one such position was a _____.
   a. noblemen   c. shaman
   b. warrior   d. tonsorial artist   ____

3. What Latin word meaning "beard" is the origin of the word *barber*?
   a. *Tondere.*   c. *Queue.*
   b. *Tonsors.*   d. *Barba.*   ____

4. During the Middle Ages, a _____ was a distinguishing style worn by clergymen.
   a. tonsure   c. mustache
   b. wig   d. queue   ____

5. Which of the following historical figures encouraged shaving by imposing a tax on beards?
   a. Alexander the Great.
   b. Peter the Great.
   c. Louis XIV.
   d. Emperor Hadrian.   ____

6. In what year did barber-surgeons begin practicing after they took over the role of physician and surgeon from the clergy?
   a. 1096.   c. 1308.
   b. 1163.   d. 1450.   ____

7. In 1540, Henry VIII recombined the barbers and surgeons of London through an Act of Parliament by granting a charter to the _____.
   a. Worshipful Company of Barbers
   b. Council of Tours
   c. Company of Barber-Surgeons
   d. Barbers' Company   ____

8. The symbol of the barber pole is thought to have evolved from what technical procedure performed by the barber-surgeons?
   a. Bloodletting.   c. Tonsorial services.
   b. Pulling teeth.   d. Cauterization.   ____

9. Many Europeans had become so dependent upon the services of the barber-surgeons that _____ settlers brought barber-surgeons with them to America.
   a. Egyptian and Greek
   b. Dutch and Swedish
   c. Italian
   d. French   ____

10. One interpretation of the red, white, and blue barber pole colors is that the colors represent _____, _____, and _____.
   a. life, water, porcelain
   b. blood, veins, bandages
   c. leaches, shaving cream, swirling colors
   d. haircutting, shaving, beard grooming   ____

11. In the early 1900s in New York City, what system outlined strict disinfection and cleaning practices?
   a. Licensed system.
   b. Workers international system.
   c. Franchise system.
   d. Terminal methods system.   ____

12. Which of the following organizations developed standards for licensing and policing the barber industry?
   a. Journeymen Barbers International Union of America.
   b. Barbers' Protective Association.
   c. National Association of Barber Boards of America (NABBA).
   d. Associated Master Barbers and Beauticians of America (AMBBA).   ____

13. The National Association of State Board of Barber
    Examiners was created in _____ to solidify required
    qualifications for barber examination applicants and the
    methods used in their evaluation.
    a. 1929   **c.** 1927
    b. 1924   **d.** 1925   ____

14. The Associated Master Barbers and Beauticians of America
    (AMBBA) adopted the *barber code of ethics* to promote

    _____.

    a. professional responsibility
    b. the profession of barbering
    c. professional education
    d. licensure   ____

15. What does the acronym NABBA stand for?
    a. National Association of State Board.
    b. National Association of Barber Code.
    c. National Association of Barber Boards of America.
    d. National Association of Barbering Bloodletting of America.   ____

16. What time period in history represented the heyday for
    American barbershops, with many men visiting their
    neighborhood shops every two weeks to maintain a clean-
    cut appearance?
    a. 1970s.   **c.** 1960s.
    b. 1940s and 1950s.   **d.** 1980s and 1990s.   ____

17. In the 1960s, the barbershop culture became less attractive
    to younger generations of men because it was associated
    with _____.
    a. the conservatism of their parents' generation
    b. the connection between the body, mind, and spirit
    c. extravagant fashion
    d. parasitic infestations   ____

18. In the 1990s, what became popular that drew men away
    from barbershops?
    a. Unisex salons.
    b. Unisex spas.
    c. Independent spas.
    d. Full-service salons and spas.   ____

3

19. One noteworthy improvement to barbering over the past century includes _____.
    a. regulatory and educational standards
    b. the restriction of types of implements available
    c. the study of psychology
    d. a relaxation of hygiene and cleaning practices   ____

20. In 2010, what barbering fashion trend returned for young men?
    a. Clean-shaven faces.
    b. Sideburns.
    c. Long hair.
    d. Beards and beard designs.   ____

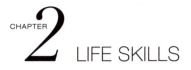

CHAPTER **2** LIFE SKILLS

MULTIPLE CHOICE

1. Approaching work with a strong sense of responsibility is considered an important _____.
   a. life skill
   b. motivation
   c. personality approach
   d. self-actualization   ____

2. A most important life skill to remember and practice is to _____.
   a. be helpful and caring toward others
   b. stick to your goals only if necessary
   c. maintain a protective attitude
   d. master techniques to become more serious and less humorous   ____

3. "I will study tomorrow instead of today" is an example of which of the following?
   a. Lack of a game plan.
   b. Visualization.
   c. Procrastination.
   d. Perfectionism.   ____

4. The process of _____ is fulfilling one's potential and requires a lifelong commitment.
   a. creativity
   b. passion
   c. self-actualization
   d. inspiration   ____

5. To create a mission statement, you must begin with your _____.
   a. confidence and self-esteem
   b. interests
   c. educational background
   d. closest friends   ____

6. The cultural pulse for organizations often comes from
   _____.
   a. the mission statement
   b. mind mapping
   c. ethics
   d. effective communication skills ____

7. Which of the following is an example of a short-term goal?
   a. Becoming a barbershop owner in 5 years.
   b. Owning your own home in 2 years.
   c. Graduating from barbering school in 6 months.
   d. Being able to retire in 6 years. ____

8. What process would you use to identify long-term and
   short-term goals?
   a. Goal setting.   c. Self-actualization.
   b. Time management.   d. Mind mapping. ____

9. When you learn to say "no" firmly but kindly, and mean it,
   you are demonstrating what time management technique?
   a. Problem solving.
   b. Prioritizing.
   c. Rewarding yourself.
   d. Not taking on more than you can handle. ____

10. Which of the following stimulates clear thinking?
    a. Repetition.
    b. Exercise and recreation.
    c. Note taking.
    d. Key words and phrases. ____

11. What time management tool helps you prioritize tasks and
    activities?
    a. Unstructured time.
    b. Physical activity.
    c. Downtime.
    d. To-do lists. ____

12. The word SHAPES, which can stand for sensation, heat
    regulation, absorption, protection, excretion, and secretion,
    is an example of _____.
    a. an acronym
    b. mind mapping
    c. word association
    d. a rhyme ____

13. When taking notes, using key words or phrases helps to identify _____.
    a. basic guidelines
    b. main points
    c. tasks and activities
    d. problem-solving techniques ____

14. If a new topic seems particularly overwhelming, what is a good way to help remember the information?
    a. Writing down the main topic.
    b. Allowing your ideas to flow.
    c. Breaking the information into smaller segments.
    d. Creating a to-do list. ____

15. When you avoid sharing clients' private matters with others, even your closest friends, you are practicing what type of behavior?
    a. Unethical.
    b. Perfectionist.
    c. Counterproductive.
    d. Ethical. ____

16. When you align your behavior and actions to your values, you are demonstrating _____.
    a. discretion   c. diplomacy
    b. integrity   d. emotional stability ____

17. An example of _____ is never breaching confidentiality by repeating personal information that clients have shared with you.
    a. discretion   c. competence
    b. sincerity   d. integrity ____

18. Being _____ is good because it helps people understand your position.
    a. critical
    b. aggressive
    c. assertive
    d. confrontational ____

19. Emotional stability plays a key part in successfully handling which of the following situations?
    a. Positive interactions.
    b. Work–life balance.
    c. Nonverbal communications.
    d. Confrontation. ____

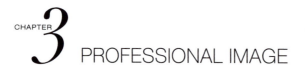

MULTIPLE CHOICE

1. Which of the following benefits the body by improving blood circulation, oxygen supply, and proper organ function?
   - **a.** Meal planning.
   - **b.** Drinking plenty of water.
   - **c.** Physical activity.
   - **d.** Relaxation. ____

2. What influence on the body can result in a series of mental and physical responses and adaptations?
   - **a.** Stress.
   - **b.** Watching television.
   - **c.** A good night's sleep.
   - **d.** A life of moderation. ____

3. The first step in maintaining good hygiene is _____.
   - **a.** using mouthwash
   - **b.** brushing your teeth
   - **c.** hand washing
   - **d.** not smoking during work hours ____

4. On average, how many hours of sleep are recommended by medical professionals?
   - **a.** 3 or 4.
   - **b.** 7 or 8.
   - **c.** 5 or 6.
   - **d.** 8 or 9. ____

5. A balanced diet includes getting plenty of _____.
   - **a.** processed foods
   - **b.** water
   - **c.** salt
   - **d.** sugar ____

6. Your professional _____ is projected through both your outward appearance and your conduct in the workplace.
   - **a.** success
   - **b.** image
   - **c.** attitude
   - **d.** health ____

7. Which of the following is of utmost importance for male barbers?
   - **a.** A barber's jacket.
   - **b.** Manicures.
   - **c.** Protective skin products.
   - **d.** Facial grooming. ____

8. Because a significant number of people are sensitive or allergic to a variety of chemicals, barbershops often have what type of policy for staff members?
   a. Stain free.
   b. Spill free.
   c. No-fragrance.
   d. Standard uniform. _____

9. A good professional choice of clothing for working in a barbershop would be clothes that are _____.
   a. pressed and clean
   b. baggy
   c. tight
   d. dirty _____

10. Wristwatches can help you stay on schedule, but it is important for them to be _____.
    a. stylish
    b. trendy
    c. waterproof
    d. flattering _____

11. Which of the following can prevent fatigue and many other physical problems?
    a. Good posture.
    b. Movement therapies.
    c. Repetitive motions.
    d. Physical therapies. _____

12. When in a stress-free standing posture behind the chair, your head should be up and your chin _____ to the floor.
    a. horizontal
    b. vertical
    c. parallel
    d. upright _____

13. When standing, your spine should be in what position?
    a. Slightly curved.
    b. Elongated.
    c. Relaxed.
    d. Straight. _____

14. What type of a motion can have a cumulative effect on the muscles and joints?
    a. Upward.
    b. Repetitive.
    c. Steady.
    d. Downward. _____

15. At what angle should your arms be positioned when holding them away from your body while working?
    a. 90 degrees.
    b. 45 degrees.
    c. 30 degrees.
    d. 60 degrees. _____

16. To avoid ergonomic-related injuries, in what position should your wrists be held?
    a. Straight or neutral.
    b. Parallel to the floor.
    c. Erect.
    d. Elongated and balanced. _____

17. To sit correctly in a balanced position, the seat of the chair should be even with your _____.
    a. hips
    b. knees
    c. spine
    d. lower parts of your arm   ____

18. What type of shoe is not safe to wear around electrical tools and sharp implements?
    a. Sneakers.
    b. Closed toed.
    c. Open toed.
    d. Boots.   ____

19. When standing behind the chair, your shoulders should be held in a(n) _____ position.
    a. level and relaxed
    b. straight
    c. elongated and balanced
    d. tilted forward or backward   ____

20. When sitting, the soles of your feet should be on the floor, directly under your _____.
    a. hips
    b. knees
    c. chair
    d. spine   ____

21. What is the key to avoiding musculoskeletal disorders in the barbering profession?
    a. Physical therapies.
    b. Movement therapies.
    c. A stress-free environment.
    d. Prevention.   ____

22. When standing to cut hair, your legs should be _____.
    a. in a stiff position
    b. bent backward
    c. hip-width apart
    d. at a 60-degree angle   ____

23. In a business setting, it is best to avoid topics such as _____.
    a. movies you have seen
    b. politics
    c. the weather
    d. sports   ____

24. What should you use when dealing with problems that you encounter?
    a. Tact.
    b. Body language.
    c. Sarcasm.
    d. Efficiency.   ____

25. Social media is a powerful tool when used correctly. You should not _____.
  a. manage your personal pages/walls
  b. forward spam
  c. post helpful content
  d. communicate with clients
  _____

26. In the barbershop, what is the first communication step to help you determine your client's service expectations?
  a. Clarify the client's needs.
  b. Organize your thoughts.
  c. Repeat the client's expectations.
  d. Establish a relationship with the client.
  _____

27. Which of the following involves establishing a close and empathetic relationship that fosters agreement and harmony between individuals?
  a. Positive attitude.   c. Confidence.
  b. Good habits.   d. Rapport.
  _____

28. What is one of the barber's most important human relations skills?
  a. Showing emotions.
  b. Projecting a certain attitude.
  c. Communication.
  d. Education.
  _____

29. Your _____ is expressed through your self-esteem and confidence and the respect you show others.
  a. professional attitude   c. capability
  b. mood   d. success
  _____

30. A desirable quality for effective client relations is that you should talk less and _____ more.
  a. respond   c. exercise
  b. listen   d. share
  _____

31. Which of the following describes the interactions and relationships between two or more people?
  a. Rapport.
  b. Empathy.
  c. Human relations.
  d. Communication.
  _____

32. What is the best way to deal with disputes or differences within the barbershop?
    a. By sharing information with others.
    b. By asking questions to gain understanding.
    c. By avoiding the topic.
    d. In private.   ____

33. As a professional, you should learn to control your emotions and respond rather than _____.
    a. disapprove
    b. react
    c. listen
    d. understand   ____

34. Establishing a professional online image is an essential _____ attribute.
    a. team camaraderie
    b. positive attitude
    c. image-building
    d. communications   ____

35. One of the benefits of effective communications skills is _____.
    a. self-promotion
    b. self-esteem
    c. self-checks
    d. self-confidence   ____

36. You should show interest in the client's personal _____.
    a. life
    b. hygiene habits
    c. preferences
    d. grooming   ____

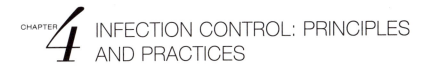

MULTIPLE CHOICE

1. Federal and state agencies regulate the practice of barbering. State agencies _____.
   a. set guidelines for use of equipment
   b. regulate licensing
   c. set guidelines for manufacturing
   d. monitor safety in the workplace ____

2. On a Safety Data Sheet, what category would include routes of exposure, related symptoms, and acute and chronic effects?
   a. Physical and chemical properties.
   b. Ecological information.
   c. Toxicology information.
   d. Stability and reactivity. ____

3. What standards address issues relating to your right to know about any potentially hazardous ingredients contained in the products and how to avoid these hazards?
   a. OSHA standards.   c. EPA standards.
   b. CDC standards.   d. SDS standards. ____

4. _____ establish specific standards of conduct and can be changed or updated frequently.
   a. Regulations   c. Statues
   b. Laws   d. Rules ____

5. Ignorance of the law is not an acceptable reason or excuse for _____.
   a. potential hazards   c. noncompliance
   b. misinformation   d. irresponsibility ____

6. What agency registers all types of disinfectants sold and used in the United States?
   a. The CDC.
   b. OSHA.
   c. U.S. Department of Labor.
   d. The EPA. ____

7. Laws are written by _____.
   a. state boards
   b. federal and state legislatures
   c. regulatory agencies
   d. health departments   ____

8. Which of the following are chemical products that destroy most bacteria, fungi, and viruses on surfaces?
   a. Disinfectants.   c. Cleansers.
   b. Sanitizers.   d. Sterilizers.   ____

9. Both federal and state laws require that manufacturers supply a(n) _____ for all chemical products manufactured and sold.
   a. Globally Harmonized System of Classification and Labeling of Chemicals System
   b. EPA list
   c. Safety Data Sheet
   d. Hazard Communication Standard   ____

10. Tuberculocidal disinfectants are often referred to as _____.
   a. nonpathogenic   c. single-use
   b. quats   d. phenolics   ____

11. Disinfection is not effective against _____.
   a. bacterial spores   c. viruses
   b. bacteria   d. molds   ____

12. What type of bacteria are harmful microorganisms that can cause disease or infection in humans when they invade the body?
   a. Nonpathogenic.   c. Infectious.
   b. Pathogenic.   d. Parasitic.   ____

13. What type of bacteria are pus-forming and grow in clusters like bunches of grapes?
   a. Cocci.   c. Staphylococci.
   b. Diplococci.   d. Streptococci.   ____

14. Diplococci are spherical bacteria that grow in pairs and cause diseases such as _____.
   a. typhoid fever   c. syphilis
   b. pneumonia   d. strep throat   ____

15. What type of bacteria rarely demonstrate self-movement and are transmitted in the air, dust, or within the substance in which they settle?
    a. Cocci.
    b. Treponema pallidum.
    c. Spirilla.
    d. Bacilli.   ____

16. A disinfectant that is a fungicidal is capable of destroying _____.
    a. parasites
    b. viruses
    c. bacteria
    d. molds   ____

17. Which of the following is a mechanical process (scrubbing) using soap and water or detergent and water?
    a. Sanitizing.
    b. Sterilizing.
    c. Cleaning.
    d. Disinfecting.   ____

18. During the inactive stage, certain bacteria can _____.
    a. grow
    b. form spores
    c. reproduce
    d. divide   ____

19. An inflammation is characterized by _____.
    a. redness, heat, pain, and/or swelling
    b. red papules or spots
    c. coughing or sneezing
    d. blood poisoning   ____

20. Which of the following are single-celled microorganisms that have both plant and animal characteristics?
    a. Fungi.
    b. Parasites.
    c. Bacteria.
    d. Viruses.   ____

21. Which of the following is capable of replication only through taking over the host cell's reproductive function?
    a. Bacteria.
    b. Viruses.
    c. Fungi.
    d. Molds.   ____

22. Staph bacteria is responsible for _____.
    a. common colds
    b. chicken pox
    c. influenza
    d. food poisoning   ____

23. A common contagious disease that would prevent a barber from servicing a client would be _____.
    a. blood poisoning
    b. Lyme disease
    c. ringworm
    d. tetanus   ____

24. When bacteria reach their largest size in the active phase, they divide into two new cells. What is this division called?
    a. Binary fission.   c. Spore-forming.
    b. Replication.   d. Distribution.   ____

25. What type of infection is it where the pathogen has distributed itself throughout the body rather than staying in one area or organ?
    a. Systemic.   c. Contagious.
    b. Communicable.   d. Local.   ____

26. All of the following are bacterial infections, that without proper treatment, can become systemic and can have devastating consequences that can result in death.
    a. AIDS.
    b. Pneumonia.
    c. Methicillin-resistant staphylococcus aureus (MRSA).
    d. Strep throat.   ____

27. One action of the biofilm community is to resist _____.
    a. pathogens and recognize infection
    b. conventional treatments such as antibiotics
    c. infection
    d. the body's defense mechanisms   ____

28. Which of the following keep the body in a chronic inflammatory state that is painful and inhibits healing?
    a. Bacterial strains.
    b. Biofilms.
    c. Contagious diseases.
    d. Communicable diseases.   ____

29. The presence of pus is a sign of a _____.
    a. bacterial infection   c. viral infection
    b. parasitic infestation d. biofilm   ____

30. Which of the following can prevent viruses from growing in the body?
    a. Virucidal disinfectant. c. Standard precautions.
    b. Antibiotics.   d. Vaccinations.   ____

31. In the barbershop, the spread of bloodborne pathogens is possible whenever _____.
    a. someone sneezes
    b. the skin is broken
    c. someone coughs
    d. you do not wash your hands   ____

32. Hepatitis is a bloodborne virus that causes disease and can damage what body organ?
    a. Kidney.   c. Heart.
    b. Lungs.   d. Liver.   ____

33. Which of the following bloodborne viruses can live on a surface outside the body for long periods of time?
    a. HIV.   c. Hepatitis.
    b. Tinea barbae.   d. AIDS.   ____

34. AIDS is a disease that breaks down the body's _____ system.
    a. immune   c. endocrine
    b. nervous   d. cardiovascular   ____

35. HIV is spread from person to person through blood and, less often, through _____.
    a. sharing food   c. body fluids
    b. holding hands   d. kissing   ____

36. HIV is spread mainly through the sharing of needles by intravenous drug users and by _____.
    a. hugging
    b. sharing food
    c. kissing
    d. unprotected sexual contact   ____

37. _____ is the process that destroys all microbial life, including spores.
    a. Sanitizing   c. Disinfecting
    b. Sterilization   d. Cleaning   ____

38. Disinfectants are _____ and can be harmful if absorbed through the skin.
    a. pesticides   c. antiseptics
    b. germicides   d. pathogens   ____

39. Effective sterilization typically requires the use of a(n)
_____.

a. countertop receptacle   **c.** heat lamp
b. UV light unit   **d.** autoclave   ____

40. The vast majority of contaminants and pathogens can be
removed from the surfaces of tools and implements through
proper _____.
a. sterilization   **c.** cleaning
b. disinfection   **d.** sanitizing   ____

41. The time as listed on the product label required for the
disinfectant to be visibly moist to be effective against
pathogens is called _____ time.
a. dilution   **c.** efficacy
b. contact   **d.** concentrate   ____

42. What should you never mix with bleach?
a. Detergents.   **c.** Disinfectants.
b. Water.   **d.** Pesticides.   ____

43. An item must remain submerged in the disinfectant for
_____ unless the product label specifies differently.
a. 2 hours   **c.** 10 minutes
b. 30 minutes   **d.** 1 hour   ____

44. Which of the following are a form of formaldehyde, have a
very high pH, and can damage the skin and eyes?
a. Petroleum distillates.
b. Quaternary ammonium compounds.
c. Bleaches.
d. Phenolic disinfectants.   ____

45. _____ are excellent at removing grime and oils from
metals.
a. Petroleum distillates
b. Phenolic disinfectants
c. Quaternary ammonium compounds
d. Bleaches   ____

46. Bleach must be stored away from _____.
a. metals and plastics
b. heat and light
c. kerosene
d. water   ____

47. Which of the following are known carcinogens?
  a. Distillates.
  c. Phenolics.
  b. Quats.
  d. Bleaches. ____

48. _____ do not disinfect or sterilize.
  a. Liquid disinfecting solutions
  c. Quats
  b. Autoclaves
  d. UV light units ____

49. Towels, linens, and capes that are not thoroughly dried may grow _____.
  a. microbes
  c. bacteria
  b. viruses
  d. parasites ____

50. Which of the following is not a disinfectant for surfaces or implements?
  a. Bleach.
  c. Phenolic disinfectants.
  b. Petroleum distillates.
  d. Alcohol. ____

51. What is one of the most important actions you can take to prevent spreading germs from one person to another?
  a. Using an antibacterial soap.
  b. Proper hand washing.
  c. Using an antimicrobial soap.
  d. Using a moisturizing hand lotion. ____

52. Antiseptics generally contain a high volume of _____.
  a. alcohol
  c. sodium hypochlorite
  b. formaldehyde
  d. ammonium ____

53. Which of the following works well as an antiseptic?
  a. Phenolics.
  b. Quaternary ammonium compounds.
  c. Hydrogen peroxide.
  d. Petroleum distillates. ____

54. A leather strop or holster is a porous material and as such cannot be _____.
  a. used multiple times
  c. cleaned
  b. heated
  d. disinfected ____

55. Which of the following can be irritating to the lungs if you inhale the fumes?
  a. Bleach.
  c. Detergents.
  b. Alcohol.
  d. Antiseptics. ____

56. Which of the following was first introduced in 1987 to reduce the spread or the transmission of bloodborne pathogens within the healthcare setting?
a. Safety Data Sheets.
b. Hazard Communication Standards.
c. Universal Precautions.
d. Standard Precautions.
_____

57. In most instances, clients who are infected with the hepatitis B virus or other bloodborne pathogens are _____.
a. symptomatic
c. not contagious
b. asymptomatic
d. under treatment
_____

58. When washing your hands, use liquid soaps in pump containers because _____ can grow in bar soaps.
a. bacteria
c. parasites
b. viruses
d. molds
_____

59. What type of incident is contact with nonintact skin, blood, body fluid, or potentially infectious materials that is the result of the performance of a worker's duties?
a. Accident.
c. Hazard.
b. Injury.
d. Exposure.
_____

60. Should you accidentally cut a client, your first action should be to _____.
a. place the razor in a container designated for cleaning and disinfection
b. wash your hands
c. stop the service immediately
d. dispose of the blade in a sharps container
_____

61. Sharp disposables should be disposed of in _____.
a. a sharps container
b. a plastic storage bag
c. a double-bagged trash bag
d. the regular trash
_____

62. At the shampoo bowl, be careful how you handle the _____.
a. water heater
c. hot-water tank
b. client's head rest
d. spray hose
_____

63. Water heaters should not be set at higher than _____ degrees Fahrenheit.
a. 100
c. 130
b. 75
d. 150
_____

64. As a precaution, you should always test the water temperature _____ before applying to a client's hair or scalp.
   a. with your fingertips
   b. on the inside of your wrist
   c. on the back of your hand
   d. on your forearm ____

65. All electrical appliances and tools should be stored safely when in proximity to _____.
   a. water
   b. the client
   c. ventilation systems
   d. air conditioners ____

66. Your clothing should be _____.
   a. tight
   b. excessively baggy
   c. comfortable
   d. loose fitting ____

67. When cutting a child's hair, how should you hold the child's head?
   a. Tightly.
   b. Loosely.
   c. With your palms only.
   d. Gently but firmly. ____

68. All employees should be instructed in _____ use.
   a. disinfectant
   b. fire extinguisher
   c. hydraulic chair
   d. implement ____

69. As a professional barber, your most important responsibility is to _____.
   a. protect your clients' health and safety
   b. keep your license current
   c. not take shortcuts for disinfecting
   d. be knowledgeable ____

70. As a professional barber, you should be aware of your environment so that you can eliminate _____.
   a. the transmission of infectious organisms
   b. pathogenic bacteria
   c. potential hazards
   d. emergencies ____

71. It is important to wear _____ while disinfecting nonelectrical tools and implements.
   a. safety glasses and gloves
   b. nonskid rubber sole shoes
   c. a gown
   d. a mask ____

72. The presence of soap in most disinfectants will cause them to become _____.

    a. harmful   **c.** inactive

    b. explosive   **d.** toxic   ____

73. Remove hair particles from clipper blades with _____.

    a. a soft brush   **c.** tongs

    b. a rubber comb   **d.** a stiff brush   ____

74. Blood may carry _____, so you should never touch an open sore or a wound.

    a. chemicals   **c.** toxic substances

    b. pathogens   **d.** potential hazards   ____

75. When handling an exposure incident, once your hands are clean you should immediately _____.

    a. stop the service

    b. put on gloves

    c. apologize for the incident

    d. clean the cut with an antiseptic   ____

76. For all of your clippers or outliners, it is important to _____ the parts regularly.

    a. aerosol spray   **c.** grease and oil

    b. sharpen   **d.** towel dry   ____

77. Before you begin cleaning a conductor cord, always double-check that it is _____.

    a. unplugged   **c.** rinsed off

    b. turned on   **d.** disinfected   ____

78. You should remove all _____ from your tools and implements before washing.

    a. contaminated objects

    b. grease or oil

    c. traces of solution or soap

    d. visible hair   ____

79. A(n) _____ is the invasion of body tissues by disease-causing pathogens.

    a. infection   **c.** disinfection

    b. contamination   **d.** fission   ____

80. Staphylococci are pus-forming bacteria that grow in
    _____.
    a. irregular masses
    b. pairs
    c. clusters like bunches of grapes
    d. strings of beads   ____

81. Pathogenic bacteria, viruses, or fungi cannot enter the body
    through which of the following?
    a. The nose.   c. Inflamed skin.
    b. Intact skin.   d. The mouth.   ____

82. _____ are poisonous substances produced by some
    microorganisms such as bacteria and viruses.
    a. Antitoxins   c. Pathogens
    b. Allergens   d. Toxins   ____

83. The CDC requires autoclaves be tested weekly to ensure
    they are properly sterilizing implements. The accepted
    method is called a _____ test.
    a. performance   c. spore
    b. steam   d. control   ____

84. On Safety Data Sheets, emergency procedures, protective
    equipment, and proper methods of containment and
    cleanup are listed as _____.
    a. accidental release measures
    b. first-aid measures
    c. exposure controls/personal protection
    d. toxicology information   ____

85. Hospital disinfectants are effective for cleaning blood and
    body fluids from _____ surfaces.
    a. environmental   c. countertop
    b. nonporous   d. porous   ____

86. The most common way contagious infections spread is
    through _____.
    a. inhalation   c. intact skin
    b. water   d. dirty hands   ____

87. The body prevents and controls infections through which of
    the following?
    a. Antitoxins.   c. Compromised skin.
    b. Taste buds.   d. Red blood cells.   ____

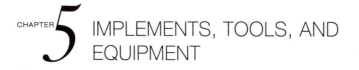 **5** IMPLEMENTS, TOOLS, AND EQUIPMENT

MULTIPLE CHOICE

1. What appliance would be used to perform finishing and styling work on your clients?
   - **a.** Razors.
   - **b.** Brushes.
   - **c.** Combs.
   - **d.** Blowdryer. ____

2. Choosing the right implement or tool for the job will depend on your understanding of the item's _____.
   - **a.** manufacturer
   - **b.** functions
   - **c.** guidelines
   - **d.** accessories ____

3. What type of combs are slightly flexible and durable but can deteriorate if left in a disinfectant over an extended time?
   - **a.** Hard rubber.
   - **b.** Graphite.
   - **c.** Metal.
   - **d.** Combs made from carbon materials. ____

4. What type of combs are preferable for detangling, creating styling effects, or distributing product through the hair?
   - **a.** Narrow-toothed.
   - **b.** Combination-toothed.
   - **c.** Wide-toothed.
   - **d.** Fine-toothed. ____

5. A _____ is an effective choice for combing through textured or tightly curled hair.
   - **a.** tail comb
   - **b.** taper comb
   - **c.** flat handle comb
   - **d.** hair pick ____

6. A round brush is used for _____.
   - **a.** creating volume
   - **b.** detangling dry hair
   - **c.** detangling wet hair
   - **d.** general drying ____

7. If you wanted a comb that was antistatic, what material would it be made from?
   - **a.** Metal.
   - **b.** Hard rubber.
   - **c.** Carbon.
   - **d.** Graphite. ____

8. Which shears are made by working heated metal into a finished shape through the processes of hammering or compression?

    a. German.   **c.** French.

    b. Forged.   **d.** Cast.   _____

9. Barbers often choose the French-style shear because _____.

    a. its disposable blade eliminates honing

    b. it facilitates shear-over-comb cutting

    c. it is less expensive

    d. the tang helps to ensure balance and control during cutting   _____

10. What type of blade consists of a convex blade that has a bevel ground onto the blade edge?

    a. Semi-convex.   **c.** Convex.

    b. Beveled edge.   **d.** Hollow ground.   _____

11. With shear blades, what part of the blade does the cutting?

    a. Point.   **c.** Cutting edge.

    b. Tang.   **d.** Shank.   _____

12. Which of the following shear parts controls the distance between the blades?

    a. Bumper.   **c.** Tension screw.

    b. Shank.   **d.** Thumb grip.   _____

13. What handle design has a shorter thumb shank to reduce overextension and is considered to be more ergonomically correct?

    a. Offset.   **c.** Angle.

    b. Opposing.   **d.** Crow.   _____

14. _____ shears create patterns and texture in hair.

    a. Texturizing   **c.** Thinning

    b. Chunking   **d.** Blending   _____

15. The finger tang is where your little finger can rest to _____.

    a. control larger amounts of hair

    b. manipulate the moving blade of the shears

    c. prevent the grips from touching when the shears are completely closed

    d. relieve pressure on your nerves and tendons   _____

16. When holding shears, do not allow the finger grip to slide past the second knuckle or you will _____.
   a. strain your arm
   b. lose control of the finger tang
   c. lose control of the shears
   d. strain your hand ____

17. When holding shears, you should insert the tip of your thumb into the thumb grip no further than your _____.
   a. second knuckle   **c.** first knuckle
   b. cuticle   **d.** the tip of your nail ____

18. You should practice opening and closing shears, using only the _____ to manipulate the moving blade of the shears.
   a. thumb   **c.** index finger
   b. little finger   **d.** wrist ____

19. Palming the shears is when the shears are closed and resting in the palm while you _____.
   a. disinfect the shears   **c.** cut the hair
   b. sharpen the shears   **d.** comb the hair ____

20. What procedure allows the first two fingers of one hand free to control the hair and the shear hand is then free to cut the hair section?
   a. Stropping the razor.
   b. Transferring and palming the comb.
   c. Honing the razor.
   d. Palming the shears. ____

21. What tool is used for finish and detail work?
   a. Adjustable-blade clippers.
   b. Metal combs.
   c. Detachable-blade clippers.
   d. Outliners. ____

22. Adjustable-blade clippers have adjustable blades that are affixed to the unit with _____.
   a. clipper guards   **c.** screws
   b. hanger loop   **d.** bumper ____

23. An electric clipper with a pivot motor would be used to cut what type of hair?
   a. Thick, coarse, or damp.   **c.** Thick and dry.
   b. All types.   **d.** Dry and fine. ____

24. In what type of electric clipper motor do the blades pull in one direction?

    a. Pivot.
    c. Rotary.
    b. Universal.
    d. Magnetic.
    ____

25. Clipper blades are usually made of high-quality carbon steel or _____.

    a. graphite
    c. hard rubber
    b. ceramic
    d. plastic
    ____

26. What are clipper guards also known as?

    a. Attachment combs.
    c. Blending shears.
    b. Hair shapers.
    d. Edgers.
    ____

27. The technique used by barbers to hold the clipper is most often determined by the _____.

    a. style of the clipper
    b. manufacturer's instructions
    c. section of the head they are working on
    d. hairstyle
    ____

28. A general rule to follow is for the barber to hold the clippers in a manner that permits _____.

    a. the closest cut
    b. uniformity within the cut
    c. faster and more precise haircutting
    d. free wrist movement
    ____

29. What is the razor of choice for professional barbering?

    a. Trimmer.
    c. Safety.
    b. Straight.
    d. Edger.
    ____

30. You should avoid judging a razor simply on _____.

    a. color or design
    b. quality
    c. other barber's recommendations
    d. manufacturer
    ____

31. What type of razor tends to be used almost exclusively in the barbershop because it helps to maintain infection control standards?

    a. Hair shaper.
    b. Conventional straight razor.
    c. Changeable-blade straight razor.
    d. Razor shaper.
    ____

32. The method for replacing the blade in a changeable-razor will vary depending on the _____.
    a. model
    b. procedure
    c. shave
    d. holding technique ____

33. If the razor handle is in a straightened position with the thumb and first two fingers almost touching at the shank, this is the technique for _____.
    a. stropping
    b. honing
    c. shaving
    d. haircutting ____

34. If the ball of the thumb and first two fingers are positioned on the flat side of the shanks with the handle pivoted up to allow the little finger to rest on the tang, this is the technique for_____.
    a. shaving
    b. honing
    c. haircutting
    d. stropping ____

35. Which of the following positions gives the most control of the razor when honing and stropping?
    a. The ball of the thumb supports the razor at the bottom of the shank and the little finger rests on the tang with the first two or three fingers at the top of the shank.
    b. The ball of the thumb and first two fingers are positioned on the flat side of the shanks with the handle pivoted up to allow the little finger to rest on the tang.
    c. The ball of the thumb and first two fingers are positioned on the flat sides of the shank with the handle in a straight position.
    d. The razor handle is in a straightened position with the thumb and first two fingers almost touching at the shank. ____

36. When a razor is properly _____, it acquires the degree of hardness required for a good cutting edge.
    a. finished
    b. balanced
    c. tempered
    d. sized ____

37. Which of the following refers to the weight and length of the blade relative to that of the handle?
    a. Razor size.
    b. Razor grind.
    c. Razor temper.
    d. Razor balance. ____

38. What is used to grind the steel and impart an effective cutting edge to the razor's blade?
    a. Temper.
    b. Strop.
    c. Hone.
    d. Grind. ____

39. A keen razor edge has fine teeth and tends to dig into a thumbnail _____.
a. without any cutting power
b. with a smooth, steady grip
c. with a jerky feeling
d. with a harsh, grating sound _____

40. The direction of the blade edge in stropping is the reverse of that used in _____.
a. honing
b. stroking
c. bracing
d. edging _____

41. What pace is preferred when stropping?
a. Slow.
b. Uneven.
c. Fast.
d. Moderate. _____

42. What type of chairs are typically smaller in design and do not usually have a head rest?
a. Motorized.
b. Hydraulic.
c. Styling.
d. Barber. _____

43. What type of towels may be preferred for shampooing and chemical services because of their absorbent qualities?
a. Synthetic.
b. Terry cloth.
c. Paper.
d. Vinyl. _____

44. _____ soap is used in electric latherizers.
a. Liquid cream
b. Soft
c. Vegetable
d. Hard _____

45. Which of the following requires the use of a stove to heat it?
a. Electric flat iron.
b. Pressing brush.
c. Electric curling iron.
d. Conventional (Marcel) iron. _____

46. What machine introduces water-soluble products into the skin during a facial?
a. Electrotherapy.
b. Tesla.
c. Galvanic.
d. High-frequency. _____

47. What method is no longer considered a safe and sanitary option for loose hair removal?
   a. Paper neck strips.
   b. Neck dusters.
   c. Vacuum systems.
   d. Paper towels. ____

48. What hair removal method may not facilitate a thorough dusting?
   a. Paper neck strips.
   b. Vacuum systems.
   c. Cloth towels.
   d. Paper towels. ____

49. What type of towel would you use for a towel wrap?
   a. Pre-steamed.
   b. Neck duster.
   c. Styling.
   d. 100 percent cotton terry cloth. ____

50. How should you grasp the towel for a towel wrap?
   a. Tautly.
   b. Loosely.
   c. Lengthwise.
   d. Vertically. ____

CHAPTER 6 GENERAL ANATOMY AND PHYSIOLOGY

MULTIPLE CHOICE

1. Which of the following is the study of the functions and activities performed by the body's structures?
   a. Osteology.
   b. Physiology.
   c. Anatomy.
   d. Histology. ____

2. The study of the human body structures seen with the naked eye and how the body parts are organized is _____.
   a. physiology
   b. histology
   c. myology
   d. anatomy ____

3. The study of tiny structures found in living tissues is known as _____.
   a. pathology
   b. physiology
   c. histology
   d. myology ____

4. What is the colorless jellylike substance found inside cells in which food elements such as proteins, fats, carbohydrates, mineral salts, and water are present?
   a. Centrioles.
   b. Cytoplasm.
   c. Plasma.
   d. Protoplasm. ____

5. What part of the cell plays an important part in cell reproduction and metabolism?
   a. Nucleus.
   b. Cell membrane.
   c. Protoplasm.
   d. Cytoplasm. ____

6. Mitosis is the usual process of cell reproduction of human tissues that occurs when the cell divides into two identical cells called _____.
   a. receptors
   b. centrioles
   c. daughter cells
   d. neurons ____

7. What part of the cell is needed for growth, reproduction, and self-repair?
   a. Protoplasm.
   b. Cytoplasm.
   c. Nucleus.
   d. Cell membrane. ____

8. What type of tissue carries messages to and from the brain and controls and coordinates all bodily functions?
   a. Epithelial.
   b. Muscle.
   c. Connective.
   d. Nerve. ____

9. An example of connective tissue is/are _____.
   a. mucous membranes
   b. skin
   c. blood
   d. the lining of the heart ____

10. Body tissues are composed of large amounts of _____.
    a. fat
    b. water
    c. minerals
    d. nutrients ____

11. What type of tissue gives smoothness and contour to the body?
    a. Nerve.
    b. Epithelial.
    c. Muscle.
    d. Adipose. ____

12. Nerve tissue is composed of special cells known as _____.
    a. microscopic cells
    b. neurons
    c. daughter cells
    d. interstitial cells ____

13. _____ are groups of body organs acting together to perform one or more functions.
    a. Body connections
    b. Body physiology
    c. Body systems
    d. Body tissues ____

14. Structures composed of specialized tissues designed to perform specific functions in plants and animals are called _____.
    a. systems
    b. nerves
    c. organs
    d. cells ____

15. _____ is the study of the anatomy, structure, and function of the bones.
    a. Osteology
    b. Pathology
    c. Histology
    d. Myology ____

16. Which of the following bones joins all of the bones of the cranium together?
    a. Parietal.
    b. Ethmoid.
    c. Sphenoid.
    d. Temporal. ____

17. What bones of the face are also known as malar bones or cheekbones?
    a. Lacrimal.
    b. Zygomatic.
    c. Mandible.
    d. Maxillae. _____

18. One of the primary functions of the skeletal system is to _____.
    a. serve as attachments for internal organs
    b. protect various external structures
    c. store most of the body's fat supply
    d. help produce white and red blood cells _____

19. What is the largest bone of the arm and extends from the shoulder to the elbow?
    a. Humerus.
    b. Ulna.
    c. Radius.
    d. Carpus. _____

20. What type of muscles are found in the internal organs of the body, such as the stomach and intestines?
    a. Voluntary.
    b. Striated (striped).
    c. Nonstriated (smooth).
    d. Cardiac. _____

21. The part of the muscle that moves and is farthest from the skeleton is the _____.
    a. origin
    b. fibrous
    c. belly
    d. insertion _____

22. What bone framework serves as a protective covering for the heart, lungs, and other delicate internal organs?
    a. Cranium.
    b. Thorax.
    c. Cervical vertebrae.
    d. Vertebral column. _____

23. Muscular tissue may be stimulated by electric current, which may be either high-frequency or _____.
    a. faradic current
    b. infrared rays
    c. steamers
    d. ultraviolet rays _____

24. The muscle that draws the scalp backward is known as the _____ muscle.
    a. epicranial aponeurosis
    b. frontalis
    c. epicranius
    d. occipitalis _____

25. What muscle is the ring muscle of the eye socket that enables you to close your eyes?
    a. Levator palpebrae superioris.
    b. Corrugator.
    c. Orbicularis oculi.
    d. Procerus. _____

26. The muscle of the mouth that draws the corner of the mouth out and back, as in grinning, is known as the _____ muscle.
    a. buccinator
    b. risorius
    c. triangularis
    d. mentalis
    ____

27. The latissimus dorsi muscle _____.
    a. helps extend the arm away from the body
    b. assists in breathing
    c. pulls the upper lip backward, upward, and outward
    d. assists the swinging movements of the arm
    ____

28. The tricep is a large muscle that _____.
    a. allows the arm to extend outward and to the side of the body
    b. lifts the forearm and flexes the elbow
    c. produces the contour of the front and inner side of the upper arm
    d. covers the entire back of the upper arm and extends the forearm
    ____

29. The muscle of the forearm that rotates the radius outward and the palm upward is the _____.
    a. pronator
    b. extensor
    c. supinator
    d. flexor
    ____

30. The muscular system covers, shapes, and supports the skeleton, and its function is to help _____.
    a. produce both white and red blood cells
    b. produce movement within the body
    c. equalize the body's temperature
    d. carry wastes and impurities away from the cells
    ____

31. An example of an immovable joint is the _____.
    a. skull
    b. hip
    c. elbow
    d. knee
    ____

32. Painful inflammation involving the carpus (wrist) area can be caused by _____.
    a. heat
    b. keeping the wrist straight
    c. prolonged standing
    d. repetitive motions
    ____

33. What body system helps regulate the body's temperature?
    a. Circulatory.
    b. Nervous.
    c. Integumentary.
    d. Lymphatic/immune.   ____

34. _____ are secretions, such as insulin, adrenaline, and estrogen, that stimulate functional activity or other secretions in the body.
    a. Hormones   c. Interstitial fluid
    b. Plasma   d. Protoplasm   ____

35. The _____ system consists of the heart, arteries, veins, and capillaries that distribute blood throughout the body.
    a. endocrine   c. respiratory
    b. circulatory   d. lymphatic/immune   ____

36. What type of glands release hormonal secretions directly into the bloodstream?
    a. Exocrine.   c. Endocrine.
    b. Hormonal.   d. Duct.   ____

37. Which of the following helps carry wastes and impurities away from the cells before it is routed back to the circulatory system?
    a. Lymph.   c. Plasma.
    b. Blood.   d. Interstitial fluid.   ____

38. The spleen is part of what body system?
    a. Reproductive.   c. Circulatory.
    b. Endocrine.   d. Lymphatic/immune.   ____

39. Cervical nerves originate at the _____.
    a. brain   c. scalp
    b. spinal cord   d. heart   ____

40. Which of the following carries blood containing waste products back to the heart and lungs for cleaning and to pick up oxygen?
    a. Veins.   c. Capillaries.
    b. Arteries.   d. Arterioles.   ____

41. Blood is approximately what percent water?
    a. 40 percent.   c. 80 percent.
    b. 50 percent.   d. 25 percent.   ____

42. In the hand, what draws the fingers together?
    a. Adductors.
    c. Abductors.
    b. Flexors.
    d. Extensors.   ____

43. What body system controls and coordinates the functions of all the other systems and makes them work harmoniously and efficiently?
    a. Respiratory.
    c. Nervous.
    b. Endocrine.
    d. Circulatory.   ____

44. Which of the following controls consciousness and all mental activities, the functions of the five senses, and voluntary muscle actions?
    a. Peripheral nervous system.
    b. Autonomic nervous system.
    c. Somatic nervous system.
    d. Central nervous system.   ____

45. Sensory nerves, also known as _____ nerves, carry impulses or messages from the sense organs to the brain.
    a. afferent
    c. efferent
    b. reflex
    d. axon   ____

46. What type of nerve supplies impulses to the upper part of the face?
    a. Infratrochlear.
    c. Ophthalmic.
    b. Maxillary.
    d. Mandibular.   ____

47. What body system passes on the genetic code from one generation to another?
    a. Lymphatic/immune system.
    c. Reproductive.
    b. Endocrine.
    d. Integumentary.   ____

48. The body system that affects the growth, development, sexual functions, and health of the entire body is the _____ system.
    a. integumentary
    c. reproductive
    b. lymphatic/immune
    d. endocrine   ____

49. One of the primary functions of the lymphatic/immune system is to _____.
    a. provide a suitable fluid environment for the cells
    b. regulate the body's temperature
    c. help produce movement within the body
    d. support the skeleton   ____

50. The brain is the part of the central nervous system contained in the _____.
  a. thorax
  c. spinal column
  b. cranium
  d. axon terminal   ____

51. Sensory nerve endings are called _____ and are located close to the surface of the skin.
  a. nodes
  c. receptors
  b. capillaries
  d. accessories   ____

52. What does the word *integument* mean?
  a. Map.
  c. Bone.
  b. Study of.
  d. Natural covering.   ____

53. Which of the following is the connection between two or more bones of the skeleton?
  a. Nerve.
  c. Joint.
  b. Tendon.
  d. Ligament.   ____

54. The _____ are the bones of the fingers, consisting of three in each finger and two in the thumb.
  a. phalanges
  c. metacarpals
  b. parietal bones
  d. temporal bones   ____

55. What body system relies upon the skeletal and nervous systems for its activities and proper operation?
  a. Circulatory.
  c. Reproductive.
  b. Muscular.
  d. Integumentary.   ____

56. The _____ system is closely connected to the cardiovascular system as they both transport streams of fluids.
  a. endocrine
  c. lymphatic/immune
  b. integumentary
  d. reproductive   ____

57. What artery supplies blood to the skin and muscles of the scalp and back of the head up to the crown?
  a. Anterior auricular.
  b. Posterior auricular.
  c. Transverse facial.
  d. Occipital.   ____

58. What color is blood when it is in the veins?
  a. Light red.
  c. Blue.
  b. Dark red.
  d. Bright red.   ____

59. What blood vessels bring nutrients to the cells and carry away waste materials?
    a. Capillaries. c. Arteries.
    b. Arterioles. d. Venules. ____

60. A normal adult heart beats about how many times per minute?
    a. 40 to 60. c. 75 to 100.
    b. 60 to 80. d. 100 to 110. ____

61. Which of the following nerves is affected during facials, primarily when you are giving a massage to your client?
    a. Trigeminal. c. Facial.
    b. Trifacial. d. Accessory. ____

62. What type of nerves carry impulses from the brain to the muscles or glands?
    a. Afferent. c. Motor.
    b. Sensory. d. Receptor. ____

63. What type of muscle is an involuntary muscle that is not duplicated anywhere else in the body?
    a. Striated. c. Nonstriated.
    b. Cardiac. d. Striped. ____

64. What bone is U-shaped and supports the tongue and its muscles?
    a. Malar. c. Mandible.
    b. Cervical vertebrae. d. Hyoid. ____

65. _____ are whitish cords made up of bundles of nerve fibers held together by connective tissue.
    a. Dendrites c. Glands
    b. Nerves d. Axons ____

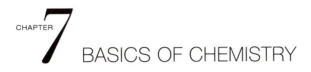

CHAPTER 7 BASICS OF CHEMISTRY

MULTIPLE CHOICE

1. What term applies to all living things and those things that were once alive?
    a. Inorganic.
    b. Matter.
    c. Organic.
    d. Element. ____

2. Gasoline, synthetic fabrics, plastics, and pesticides are all considered organic because they are manufactured from

    _____.
    a. natural gas and oil
    b. subatomic particles
    c. sodium chloride
    d. ammonium thioglycolate acid ____

3. Metals, minerals, water, air, and ammonia are all examples of _____ substances.
    a. live
    b. inorganic
    c. natural
    d. organic ____

4. Organic chemistry is the study of substances that contain the element _____.
    a. oxygen
    b. hydrogen
    c. sulfur
    d. carbon ____

5. Which of the following is defined as anything that occupies space (volume) and has mass (weight)?
    a. Atoms.
    b. Molecules.
    c. Matter.
    d. Elements. ____

6. There are 118 different elements known to science today. How many of these are naturally occurring on Earth?
    a. 116.
    b. 98.
    c. 50.
    d. 76. ____

7. Which of the following are the basic building blocks of all matter?
    a. Electrons.
    b. Protons.
    c. Molecules.
    d. Atoms. ____

8. _____ is the most common element found in the known universe.
    a. Hydrogen   **c.** Carbon dioxide
    b. Oxygen   **d.** Sodium   ____

9. An example of an elemental molecule is _____.
    a. hydrogen peroxide
    b. common table salt
    c. water
    d. the oxygen in air   ____

10. As the basic unit of matter, _____ cannot be divided into simpler substances by ordinary chemical means.
    a. molecules   **c.** atoms
    b. oxygen   **d.** water   ____

11. Rusting iron and burning wood are examples of a change in what type of properties?
    a. Chemical.   **c.** Mechanical.
    b. Physical.   **d.** Electrical.   ____

12. What chemical compound can exist in all three states of matter depending on its temperature?
    a. Carbon dioxide.   **c.** Water.
    b. Hydrogen.   **d.** Oxygen.   ____

13. An example of physical change is _____.
    a. rusting iron   **c.** burning wood
    b. ice melting to water   **d.** oxidation   ____

14. In hair lightening processes, what substance oxidizes the melanin pigments in hair, leaving the hair a lighter color?
    a. Sodium chloride.
    b. Water.
    c. Ammonium thioglycolate acid.
    d. Hydrogen peroxide.   ____

15. An example of a chemical change is _____.
    a. water changing to ice
    b. ice melting to water
    c. the oxidation of haircolor products
    d. temporary haircolor   ____

16. _____ refers to either the loss of oxygen or the addition of hydrogen.
- **a.** Application.
- **b.** Reduction.
- **c.** Reaction.
- **d.** Oxidation.

_____

17. When using a permanent wave neutralizer, _____.
- **a.** H_2O_2 loses oxygen
- **b.** the waving solution is oxidized
- **c.** haircolor gains oxygen from H_2O_2
- **d.** hair is oxidized by removing hydrogen

_____

18. When oxygen is combined with a substance, the substance is _____.
- **a.** oxidized
- **b.** reduced
- **c.** united
- **d.** blended

_____

19. Oxidation and reduction always occur simultaneously and are referred to as a(n) _____ reaction.
- **a.** rapid oxidation
- **b.** endothermic
- **c.** redox
- **d.** exothermic

_____

20. What type of chemical reaction requires the absorption of energy or heat from an external source for the reaction to actually occur?
- **a.** Endothermic.
- **b.** Acid–alkali neutralization.
- **c.** Exothermic.
- **d.** Redox.

_____

21. Which of the following is an example of a pure substance?
- **a.** Concrete.
- **b.** Aluminum foil.
- **c.** Powder.
- **d.** Salt water solution.

_____

22. _____, also known as alkalis, are compounds of hydrogen, a metal, and oxygen.
- **a.** Oxides
- **b.** Salts
- **c.** Acids
- **d.** Bases

_____

23. What color do acids turn blue litmus paper?
- **a.** A darker blue.
- **b.** Red.
- **c.** Green.
- **d.** Yellow.

_____

24. A _____ is a stable, uniform mixture of two or more mixable substances that is made by dissolving a solid, liquid, or gaseous substance in another substance.
a. suspension   **c.** solution
b. solvent   **d.** solute   ____

25. Which of the following allows oil and water to mix or emulsify by reducing surface tension?
a. Surfactant.   **c.** Emulsion.
b. Suspension.   **d.** Solution.   ____

26. An example of a water-in-oil emulsion is _____.
a. calamine lotion   **c.** witch hazel
b. mayonnaise   **d.** cold cream   ____

27. _____ are examples of emulsions used in barbering services.
a. Powders
b. Shampoos and conditioners
c. Hair tonics
d. Soaps   ____

28. A(n) _____ is a suspension of one liquid dispersed in another.
a. emulsion   **c.** solution
b. surfactant   **d.** solvent   ____

29. A(n) _____ charged ion is called an anion.
a. positively   **c.** negatively
b. ionized   **d.** naturally   ____

30. The pH scale measures the concentration of hydrogen ions in acidic and alkaline _____ solutions.
a. unstable   **c.** liquid
b. hydrogen peroxide   **d.** water-based   ____

31. What does a pH below 7 indicate?
a. A logarithmic solution.   **c.** An acidic solution.
b. An alkaline solution.   **d.** A neutral solution.   ____

32. The letters pH denote _____, which is the relative degree of acidity or alkalinity of a substance.
a. potential hydrogen
b. potential hydroxide
c. partial hydrogen
d. partially hydrophilic   ____

33. Nonaqueous solutions, such as alcohol or oil, do not have
_____.

    a. mass

    b. pH

    c. their own distinct physical and chemical properties

    d. volume or shape   ____

34. What is the average pH for hair and skin?

    a. 3.5.   **c.** 7.5.

    b. 9.   **d.** 5.   ____

35. Acidic solutions tend to _____ the hair.

    a. swell   **c.** soften

    b. harden   **d.** relax   ____

36. Acid-balanced shampoos and normalizing lotions
associated with hydroxide hair relaxers work to create what
type of reaction?

    a. Endothermic.

    b. Exothermic.

    c. Acid–alkali neutralization.

    d. Redox.   ____

37. What common cationic ingredient is used in dandruff
shampoos?

    a. Cocamide.

    b. Amphoteric I-20.

    c. Quaternary ammonium compounds.

    d. Sodium laureth sulfate.   ____

38. What type of shampoos are mild formulations designed to
prevent the stripping of haircolor from the hair?

    a. pH-balanced.   **c.** Balancing.

    b. Clarifying.   **d.** Color-enhancing.   ____

39. _____ shampoos are formulated to make the hair
smooth and shiny and to avoid damaging chemically treated
hair.

    a. Balancing   **c.** Medicated

    b. Conditioning   **d.** Clarifying   ____

40. An example of an instant conditioner is a _____.

    a. blow drying spray

    b. permanent wave product

    c. detangling rinse

    d. dandruff rinse   ____

41. Which of the following are chemical compounds that attract and retain moisture from the atmosphere?
   a. Silicones.
   c. Mineral oils.
   b. Fatty alcohols.
   d. Humectants.
   _____

42. What products are used to stimulate the surface circulation of the scalp, remove loose dandruff, or to impart manageability, shine, and control to the hair?
   a. Thermal protectors.
   b. Hair tonics.
   c. Medicated conditioners.
   d. Instant conditioners.
   _____

43. Concentrated protein conditioners are used to _____.
   a. increase the tensile strength of the hair
   b. help control minor dandruff and scalp conditions
   c. help equalize the porosity of the hair shaft
   d. help close the cuticle scales
   _____

44. Which of the following remove hair by pulling it out of the follicle?
   a. Packs.
   c. Epilators.
   b. Masks.
   d. Depilatories.
   _____

45. Styling aids typically consist of polymer and resin formulations that are designed to give the hair body and texture. An example is _____.
   a. mousses
   c. pomades
   b. scalp lotions
   d. cleansing creams
   _____

46. Among the possible ingredients in wrinkle treatment creams are hormones and _____.
   a. hydrolyzed protein
   c. starch
   b. glycerin
   d. collagen
   _____

47. Astringents may have an alcohol content of up to what percentage?
   a. 50 percent.
   c. 35 percent.
   b. 15 percent.
   d. 20 percent.
   _____

48. Moisturizing creams are designed to treat _____.
   a. oil accumulation
   c. dandruff
   b. dryness
   d. wrinkles
   _____

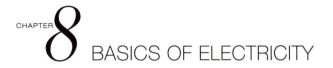

CHAPTER **8** BASICS OF ELECTRICITY

MULTIPLE CHOICE

1. Improperly repaired tools and appliances can result in
   _____.
   a. electrical pressure
   b. blown circuit breakers
   c. twisted metal threads
   d. alternating current ____

2. A(n) _____ is the flow of electricity along a conductor.
   a. rheostat   c. electric current
   b. insulator   d. electric circuit ____

3. Electricity is a form of energy created by the flow of
   electrons between _____.
   a. atoms   c. salts
   b. acids   d. metals ____

4. Electricity is not matter because it does not _____.
   a. control the current in a circuit
   b. produce a chemical reaction
   c. move through or across matter and space
   d. occupy space or have mass ____

5. Which of the following can move through or across matter
   and space?
   a. Ultraviolet light.
   b. Electricity.
   c. Light-emitting diodes.
   d. Electromagnetic radiation. ____

6. A(n) _____ is an adjustable resistor that is used for
   controlling the current in a circuit.
   a. rectifier
   b. insulator
   c. rheostat
   d. battery-operated instrument ____

7. Which of the following is considered a good conductor?
   a. Rubber.
   b. Cement.
   c. Silk.
   d. Watery solutions of acids and salts.   ____

8. What does the volt measure?
   a. Electrical pressure.
   b. Strength or rate of an electric current.
   c. Electrical resistance.
   d. How much electric energy is being used in 1 second.   ____

9. The electricity in a house is measured in _____.
   a. amperes   c. milliamperes
   b. kilowatt-hours   d. ohms   ____

10. What safety device prevents the overheating of electrical
    wires by preventing excessive current from passing through
    a circuit?
    a. Three-prong plug.   c. Fuse.
    b. Ground fault interrupter. d. Circuit breaker.   ____

11. In modern electric circuits, which of the following has
    replaced fuses and can be reset?
    a. Circuit breakers.
    b. Adjustable resistors.
    c. Rectifiers.
    d. Ground fault interrupters.   ____

12. All electrical appliances must have at least two electrical
    connections. One connection is _____ and the other is
    _____.
    a. hot; cold   c. live; hot
    b. neutral; cold   d. neutral; live   ____

13. How should you disconnect an appliance?
    a. By pulling on the cord.
    b. By stepping on the cord.
    c. By pulling on the plug.
    d. By twisting the plug.   ____

14. Which of the following should you not touch while using an
    electrical appliance?
    a. Rubber.   c. Glass.
    b. Plastic.   d. Metal.   ____

15. _____ indicates the negative or positive pole of an electric current.

a. Activity

b. Polarity

c. Elasticity

d. Modality _____

16. What type of current is a DC, using a negative and positive pole, that is reduced to a safe, low-voltage level?

a. High-frequency.

b. Microcurrent also add.

c. Tesla.

d. Galvanic. _____

17. What process introduces water-soluble products into the skin?

a. Iontophoresis.

b. Desincrustation.

c. Cataphoresis.

d. Anaphoresis. _____

18. During what process is galvanic current used to create a chemical reaction that acts to emulsify the sebum and waste in the pores?

a. Cataphoresis.

b. Anaphoresis.

c. Desincrustation.

d. Iontophoresis. _____

19. What effect can microcurrents produce?

a. Decrease muscle tone.

b. Produce a softer appearance to aging skin.

c. Decrease metabolism.

d. Restore elasticity. _____

20. What current is commonly called the _violet ray_ and is used for both scalp and facial treatments?

a. Electrotherapy.

b. Galvanic.

c. Tesla high-frequency.

d. Microcurrent. _____

21. Gamma rays are used _____.

a. for nuclear power plants

b. by physicians and dentists

c. for light-therapy services

d. in microwave ovens _____

22. Which light rays are used in ultraviolet germicidal irradiation to inactivate or destroy microorganisms?

a. Visible light.

b. UVB rays.

c. UVC rays.

d. Infrared light. _____

23. In the field of barbering, we are concerned with the invisible rays found at the two ends of the visible spectrum of light: infrared rays, which produce heat, and ultraviolet rays, which produce _____.
   a. chemical and germicidal reactions
   b. mechanical actions
   c. electric current
   d. magnetic reactions   ____

24. Within the visible spectrum of light, _____ has the shortest wavelength and _____ has the longest.
   a. yellow; red   c. yellow; green
   b. violet; red   d. violet; indigo   ____

25. What light is also known as cold light or actinic light?
   a. Electromagnetic.   c. Infrared.
   b. Visible.   d. Ultraviolet.   ____

26. What medical device is used to reduce acne, increase skin circulation, and improve collagen content in the skin?
   a. Selective photothermolysis.
   b. Therapeutic lamp.
   c. Light-emitting diode.
   d. Laser.   ____

27. When using LEDs, what color light reduces acne and bacteria?
   a. Blue.   c. Yellow.
   b. Red.   d. Green.   ____

28. When using therapeutic bulbs, what light can be used to treat acne, tinea, seborrhea, and dandruff conditions?
   a. White.   c. Blue.
   b. Ultraviolet.   d. Red.   ____

29. What medical device is designed to deliver an intense light beam to a specific depth and to a specific target area without damaging the surrounding tissues?
   a. Light-emitting diodes.   c. Therapeutic lamps.
   b. Microwave.   d. Laser.   ____

30. The client's _____ should always be protected during light-therapy treatments.
   a. ears.   c. eyes.
   b. hair.   d. skin.   ____

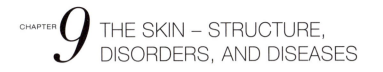

9 THE SKIN – STRUCTURE, DISORDERS, AND DISEASES

MULTIPLE CHOICE

1. On what part of the body is the skin the thinnest?
   - **a.** Shoulders.
   - **b.** Eyelids.
   - **c.** Scalp.
   - **d.** Hands. _____

2. Which of the following is the outer layer of the epidermis?
   - **a.** Stratum granulosum.
   - **b.** Stratum spinosum.
   - **c.** Stratum corneum.
   - **d.** Stratum lucidum. _____

3. The epidermis contains no _____, but has many small nerve endings.
   - **a.** melanin
   - **b.** keratin
   - **c.** fibrous protein
   - **d.** blood vessels _____

4. What epidermis layer is responsible for the growth of the epidermis?
   - **a.** Stratum germinativum.
   - **b.** Stratum corneum.
   - **c.** Stratum granulosum.
   - **d.** Stratum spinosum. _____

5. Subcutaneous tissue, also known as _____ tissue, is a layer of fatty tissue found below the dermis.
   - **a.** elastic
   - **b.** fibrous
   - **c.** adipose
   - **d.** connective _____

6. What substance lubricates the skin and preserves the softness of the hair?
   - **a.** Collagen.
   - **b.** Melanin.
   - **c.** Elastin.
   - **d.** Sebum. _____

7. Which nerve fibers carry impulses from the brain to control muscle movement?
   - **a.** Secretory.
   - **b.** Sensory.
   - **c.** Motor.
   - **d.** Receptor. _____

8. What layer of the dermis contains the lymph glands?
   - **a.** Reticular.
   - **b.** Basal cell.
   - **c.** Granular.
   - **d.** Papillary. _____

9. _____ supply nourishment to the skin in the form of protein, carbohydrates, and fat.
   a. Sebum and lymph
   c. Water and oxygen
   b. Blood and lymph
   d. Blood and water
   _____

10. What can occur to the skin when collagen fibers become weakened?
   a. Wrinkles and sagging of the skin.
   b. Skin tags.
   c. Fatty tissue.
   d. Goose bumps.
   _____

11. The color of the skin, whether fair or dark, depends on genetics and _____.
   a. sebum
   c. melanin
   b. keratin
   d. collagen
   _____

12. One of the most prominent characteristics of aged skin is its _____.
   a. formation of blackheads
   c. loss of color
   b. oiliness
   d. loss of elasticity
   _____

13. What body system controls the activity of sweat glands, which regulate body temperature and help to eliminate waste products from the body?
   a. Circulatory.
   c. Endocrine.
   b. Nervous.
   d. Lymphatic/immune.
   _____

14. The outermost layer of the epidermis is covered with a thin layer of sebum, which makes skin _____.
   a. waterproof
   c. absorbent
   b. taut
   d. sensitive
   _____

15. What is sebum secretion affected by?
   a. Injury.
   c. Heat.
   b. Pathogens.
   d. Hormones.
   _____

16. How much do humans perspire daily?
   a. 1 gallon.
   c. 1 to 2 pints.
   b. 1 to 2 cups.
   d. 1 to 2 quarts.
   _____

17. _____ is a function of the skin that protects the body from the environment.
   a. Secretion
   c. Absorption
   b. Heat regulation
   d. Excretion
   _____

18. The skin protects the body from injury and _____.
   a. pain   **c.** pathogens
   b. pressure   **d.** emotional stress   ____

19. A _____ is a small blister or sac containing clear fluid, lying within or just beneath the epidermis.
   a. tumor   **c.** macule
   b. nodule   **d.** vesicle   ____

20. An example of a bulla is _____.
   a. impetigo   **c.** lipoma
   b. severe acne   **d.** a liver spot   ____

21. Which of the following primary lesions requires a medical referral?
   a. Macule.   **c.** Papule.
   b. Cyst.   **d.** Pustule.   ____

22. A wheal can be caused by _____.
   a. acne   **c.** a mosquito bite
   b. poison ivy   **d.** second degree burns ____

23. An abnormal mass varying in size, shape, and color is a _____.
   a. tumor   **c.** bulla
   b. cyst   **d.** nodule   ____

24. Severely cracked or chapped hands or lips is considered a(n) _____.
   a. ulcer   **c.** fissure
   b. crust   **d.** keloid   ____

25. An excoriation could be caused by _____.
   a. chicken pox
   b. psoriasis
   c. a post-operative repair
   d. nail biting   ____

26. Which of the following is a thick scar resulting from excessive growth of fibrous tissue?
   a. Excoriation.   **c.** Cicatrix.
   b. Keloid.   **d.** Crust.   ____

27. What type of lesions are characterized by an accumulation of material on the skin surface or by depressions in the skin surface?

    a. Secondary.   **c.** Primary.

    b. Minor.   **d.** Major.   ____

28. Psoriasis is characterized by a(n) _____.

    a. accumulation of sebum and pus

    b. thin, dry, or oily plate of epidermal flakes

    c. crack in the skin that penetrates the dermis

    d. open lesion on the skin or mucous membrane   ____

29. Which of the following is a recurring viral infection that produces fever blisters or cold sores characterized by a single vesicle or group of vesicles with red, swollen bases?

    a. Psoriasis.   **c.** Herpes simplex I.

    b. Eczema.   **d.** Ivy dermatitis.   ____

30. _____ occurs when irritating substances, such as chemicals or tints, temporarily damage the epidermis.

    a. Irritant contact dermatitis   **c.** Psoriasis

    b. Eczema   **d.** Herpes simplex II   ____

31. Which of the following conditions may spread to other parts of the body by contact with contaminated hands, clothing, or objects?

    a. Irritant contact dermatitis.   **c.** Eczema.

    b. Ivy dermatitis.   **d.** Dermatitis.   ____

32. _____ usually occurs on the scalp, elbows, knees, chest, or lower back, but rarely on the face.

    a. Eczema   **c.** Herpes simplex II

    b. Herpes simplex I   **d.** Psoriasis   ____

33. Dermatitis lesions may appear in various forms, such as _____.

    a. wheals   **c.** vesicles

    b. fissures   **d.** nodules   ____

34. Excessive oiliness on the skin or scalp may indicate the presence of _____.

    a. milia   **c.** rosacea

    b. telangiectasis   **d.** seborrhea   ____

35. Which of the following disorders of the sebaceous glands is commonly associated with newborn babies?
a. Seborrhea.
b. Milia.
c. Open comedo.
d. Whitehead.
____

36. What disorder of the sudoriferous glands can be life threatening and requires medical attention?
a. Anhidrosis.
b. Bromhidrosis.
c. Hyperhidrosis.
d. Miliaria rubra.
____

37. _____ results in foul-smelling perspiration, usually noticeable in the armpits or on the feet.
a. Hyperhidrosis
b. Miliaria rubra
c. Bromhidrosis
d. Anhidrosis
____

38. What disorder of the sudoriferous glands is caused by exposure to excessive heat and usually clears in a short time without treatment?
a. Bromhidrosis.
b. Hyperhidrosis.
c. Anhidrosis.
d. Miliaria rubra.
____

39. What is the technical term for freckles?
a. Vitiligo.
b. Lentigines.
c. Leukoderma.
d. Hypopigmentation.
____

40. An absence of melanin pigment in the body, including the skin, hair, and eyes, is known as _____.
a. albinism
b. leukoderma
c. hyperpigmentation
d. chloasma
____

41. Which of the following changes in the pigmentation of the skin is commonly referred to as liver spots in older adults?
a. Chloasma.
b. Leukoderma.
c. Lentigines.
d. Nevus.
____

42. _____ is caused by a burn, scar, inflammation, or congenital disease that destroys the pigment-producing cells.
a. Lentigines
b. Vitiligo
c. Albinism
d. Leukoderma
____

43. Skin with vitiligo must be _____.
a. protected from overexposure to the sun
b. exposed to sunlight and air
c. exfoliated or treated by a dermatologist
d. treated with antibiotics
____

44. Which of the following is also known as a birthmark?

   a. Stain.   **c.** Chloasma.

   b. Nevus.   **d.** Vitiligo.   ____

45. A callus is a _____ that is caused by continued, repeated pressure or friction on any part of the skin.

   a. chloasma   **c.** keratoma

   b. verruca   **d.** leukoderma   ____

46. Any change in a mole requires _____.

   a. removal

   b. exfoliation

   c. protection from overexposure of the sun

   d. medical attention   ____

47. Which of the following is caused by a virus and is infectious?

   a. Mole.   **c.** Skin tag.

   b. Wart.   **d.** Keratoma.   ____

48. _____ can spread from one location to another, particularly along a scratch in the skin.

   a. Verruca   **c.** Leukoderma

   b. Vitiligo   **d.** Hypopigmentation   ____

49. If the thickening of a callus grows inward, it is called a _____.

   a. verruca   **c.** corn

   b. wart   **d.** blemish   ____

50. Where do skin tags most frequently occur?

   a. Face.   **c.** Hands and feet.

   b. Neck and chest.   **d.** Scalp.   ____

51. The most common and least severe skin cancer is _____.

   a. basal cell carcinoma

   b. basal cell melanoma

   c. squamous cell carcinoma

   d. malignant melanoma   ____

52. What type of skin cancer is characterized by black or dark brown patches on the skin that may appear uneven in texture, jagged, or raised?

   a. Squamous cell melanoma.

   b. Basal cell carcinoma.

   c. Malignant melanoma.

   d. Squamous cell carcinoma.   ____

53. The American Cancer Society recommends using the ABCDE Cancer Checklist to help make potential skin cancer easier to recognize. What does the "D" stand for in this acronym?
    a. Diagnosis.
    b. Duration.
    c. Distance.
    d. Diameter. _____

54. What vitamin is important to skin and tissue repair?
    a. D.
    b. C.
    c. A.
    d. E. _____

55. Vitamin E _____.
    a. promotes healthy and rapid healing of the skin
    b. supports the overall health of the skin
    c. helps to fight against the harmful effects of the sun's rays
    d. is important to skin and tissue repair _____

56. The American Cancer Society recommends using the ABCDE Cancer Checklist to help make potential skin cancer easier to recognize. What does the "C" stand for in this acronym?
    a. Character.
    b. Color.
    c. Cause.
    d. Consistency. _____

57. Basal cell carcinoma has what percentage of a survival rate with early diagnosis and treatment?
    a. 90%.
    b. 62%.
    c. 94%.
    d. 100%. _____

58. Which of the following skin cancers is the least common of the cancers, but is 100 percent fatal if left untreated?
    a. Squamous cell melanoma.
    b. Squamous cell carcinoma.
    c. Basal cell carcinoma.
    d. Malignant melanoma. _____

59. Early detection and treatment of malignant melanoma can result in a 94 percent 5-year survival rate, which drops drastically, to 62 percent, once it reaches the _____.
    a. lymph nodes
    b. scalp
    c. mucous membranes
    d. fibrous tissue _____

60. Using sunscreen with an _____ when in the sun is necessary to protect the skin.
    a. SPF 15
    b. SPF 30
    c. SPF 80
    d. SPF 100 _____

61. _____ and protection are the major factors involved in maintaining the skin's overall health and appearance.
    a. Seeing a dermatologist   **c.** Diet
    b. Medical treatment   **d.** Diagnosis   ____

62. Which of the following is a small brownish spot or blemish on the skin, ranging in color from pale tan to brown or bluish black?
    a. Mole.   **c.** Skin tag.
    b. Wart.   **d.** Verruca.   ____

63. The change in pigmentation of skin caused by exposure to the sun or ultraviolet light is a _____.
    a. nevus   **c.** leukoderma
    b. stain   **d.** tan   ____

64. Characteristics of _____ include eyes that are pink, and skin that is sensitive to light and ages early.
    a. lentigines   **c.** hyperpigmentation
    b. albinism   **d.** vitiligo   ____

65. Which of the following are irregularly shaped dark spots, sometimes found on the scalp and ears and often first detected by a barber?
    a. Melanomas.   **c.** Milias.
    b. Sebaceous cysts.   **d.** Open comedos.   ____

66. Sores that do not heal or unexpected skin bleeding may be symptoms of _____.
    a. disorders of the sudoriferous glands
    b. hypertrophies
    c. skin cancer
    d. dyschromias   ____

CHAPTER 10 PROPERTIES AND DISORDERS OF THE HAIR AND SCALP

MULTIPLE CHOICE

1. Which of the following is the tube-like depression or pocket in the skin or scalp that contains the hair root?
   - **a.** Arrector pili.
   - **b.** Hair follicle.
   - **c.** Dermal papilla.
   - **d.** Hair bulb. ____

2. The lower part of the hair bulb is hollow and fits over and covers the _____.
   - **a.** dermal papilla
   - **b.** endocrine glands
   - **c.** arrector pili
   - **d.** sebaceous glands ____

3. Which of the following contains the blood and nerve supply that provides the nutrients needed for hair growth?
   - **a.** Dermal papilla.
   - **b.** Arrector pili.
   - **c.** Cortex.
   - **d.** Medulla. ____

4. Overactive sebaceous glands that secrete too much sebum can cause what type of scalp condition?
   - **a.** Scale-like.
   - **b.** Dry.
   - **c.** Oily.
   - **d.** Flakey. ____

5. Hair follicles are distributed all over the body, with the exception of the palms of the hands and the _____.
   - **a.** fingers
   - **b.** top of the feet
   - **c.** ears
   - **d.** soles of the feet ____

6. The outermost layer of the hair is the _____.
   - **a.** cortex
   - **b.** follicle
   - **c.** cuticle
   - **d.** medulla ____

7. What percentage of the total weight of the hair comes from the cortex?
   - **a.** Less than 10 percent.
   - **b.** 90 percent.
   - **c.** 51 percent.
   - **d.** 40 percent. ____

8. What layer of hair may be absent in very fine and naturally blond hair?
   - **a.** Medulla.
   - **b.** Cuticle.
   - **c.** Cortex.
   - **d.** Keratin. ____

9. A healthy, compact cuticle layer is responsible for the _____ of the hair.
   a. waviness   c. color
   b. thickness   d. shine and silkiness   ____

10. The cortex's unique _____ provides strength, elasticity, and natural color to the hair.
   a. pigment   c. texture
   b. protein structure d. chemical composition   ____

11. Protein is made of chemical units called _____.
   a. hydroxids   c. amino acids
   b. pH   d. disulfides   ____

12. The hair shaft is a nonliving fiber composed of _____.
   a. sebum   c. round cells
   b. melanin pigment   d. keratinized protein   ____

13. The spiral shape of a coiled protein is called a _____.
   a. helix   c. bond
   b. chain   d. cysteine   ____

14. What type of a side bond is a weak, physical, cross-link side bond that is easily broken by water or heat?
   a. Oxygen.   c. Hydrogen.
   b. Disulfide.   d. Salt.   ____

15. A salt bond is a weak, physical side bond, which cross-links the polypeptide chains, but it reacts to changes in _____.
   a. pH   c. temperature
   b. hormones   d. oxidation   ____

16. Disulfide bonds are broken by _____.
   a. heat   c. chemical relaxers
   b. water   d. pH   ____

17. Natural hair color is the result of the _____ found within the cortex.
   a. COHNS elements
   b. amino acids
   c. chemical cross bonds
   d. melanin pigment   ____

18. Natural hair wave patterns are the result of _____.
    a. hormonal changes   c. age
    b. genetics   d. melanin pigment   ____

19. What type of hair often has low elasticity, breaks easily, and has a tendency to knot, especially on the ends?
    a. Extremely curly.   c. Wavy.
    b. Extremely straight.   d. Curly.   ____

20. The more disulfide bonds in the hair, the more resistant it will be to _____.
    a. turning gray   c. daily hair loss
    b. detangling   d. chemical processes   ____

21. During what cycle of hair growth is new hair grown?
    a. Anagen.   c. Telogen.
    b. Androgen.   d. Catagen.   ____

22. A _____ is a tuft of hair that stands straight up.
    a. vellus   c. cowlick
    b. hair stream   d. whorl   ____

23. What type of hair is the long, coarse hair found on the scalp, legs, arms, and bodies of males and females?
    a. Vellus.   c. Medulla.
    b. Lanugo.   d. Terminal.   ____

24. What is the average growth rate of healthy hair on the scalp per month?
    a. 1¼ inches.   c. 1 inch.
    b. ½ inch.   d. 1½ inches.   ____

25. Which of the following has been scientifically proven to increase hair growth?
    a. Singeing.
    b. Finasteride.
    c. Scalp massage.
    d. Application of ointments or oils.   ____

26. When two hair streams slope in opposite directions, they form _____.
    a. cowlicks
    b. whorls
    c. a natural part in the hair
    d. bald spots   ____

27. Gray hair is the same as pigmented hair except for
_____.
   a. the lack of pigment
   b. the varying degrees of curl
   c. it may grow back more evenly
   d. the angle at which the hair emerges from the hair follicle   ____

28. How often are eyebrow hairs and eyelashes replaced?
   a. Every 6 months.   c. 75 to 100 days.
   b. 1 to 2 months.   d. Every 4 to 5 months.   ____

29. During what hair growth phase does the follicle shrink,
the hair bulb disappear, and the shrunken root end form a
rounded club?
   a. Anagen.   c. Telogen.
   b. Catagen.   d. Androgen.   ____

30. Scalp massages _____.
   a. increase hair growth
   b. make hair grow back more evenly
   c. increase blood circulation
   d. make hair grow back faster   ____

31. Which of the following is an autoimmune disorder that
causes the affected hair follicles to be mistakenly attacked
by the person's own immune system?
   a. Alopecia areata.   c. Androgenic alopecia.
   b. Alopecia prematura.   d. Alopecia totalis.   ____

32. What type of alopecia is male pattern baldness, which
usually progresses to the familiar horseshoe-shaped fringe
of hair?
   a. Alopecia senilis.   c. Androgenic alopecia.
   b. Alopecia universalis.   d. Alopecia premature.   ____

33. A sensitive topic that you can speak to your client about is:
   a. marital problems.
   b. mental health concerns.
   c. money problems.
   d. abnormal hair loss.   ____

34. Almost 40 percent of men and women show some degree of hair loss by what age?

a. 35.
c. In their teens.
b. 40.
d. 63. ____

35. Clients who exhibit symptoms of _____ should be referred to a physician.

a. alopecia senilis
c. alopecia prematura
b. alopecia areata
d. androgenic alopecia ____

36. Which of the following is a topical treatment that has been proven to stimulate hair growth?

a. Minoxidil.
c. Propecia.
b. Malassezia.
d. Finasteride. ____

37. A side effect of finasteride is _____.

a. weight loss
b. further hair loss
c. loss of sexual function
d. a rash ____

38. Acquired canities develops with age and is the result of _____.

a. poor nutrition
c. a fungus
b. previous over-processing
d. genetics ____

39. Which of the following is a condition of abnormal growth of hair?

a. Canities.
c. Trichoptilosis.
b. Hypertrichosis.
d. Trichorrhexis nodosa. ____

40. Monilethrix is the technical term for _____.

a. brittle hair
c. knotted hair
b. beaded hair
d. split ends ____

41. The only way to remove split ends is to _____.

a. soften the hair with moisturizers
b. treat with hair conditioners
c. treat with scalp conditioner
d. cut them ____

42. Tinea is the medical term for _____.

a. head lice
c. ringworm
b. dandruff
d. folliculitis ____

43. What is a characteristic of scabies?
    a. Excessive itching.
    b. Musty odor.
    c. Dry, sulfur-yellow, cuplike crusts.
    d. Brittle hair. _____

44. Classic dandruff is characterized by _____.
    a. an accumulation of greasy or waxy scales
    b. a small, reddened patch of little blisters
    c. scalp irritation and large flakes
    d. red papules or spots _____

45. Tinea barbae is a superficial fungal infection caused by dermatophytes occurring chiefly over the _____.
    a. top of the scalp   c. nape of the neckline
    b. bearded area of the face   d. entire scalp _____

46. _____ is a chronic bacterial infection involving the areas surrounding the follicles of the beard and mustache areas.
    a. A furuncle
    b. Folliculitis barbae
    c. Pseudofolliculitis barbae
    d. Sycosis vulgaris _____

47. Which of the following can be caused by improper shaving or by broken hair below the skin surface that grows into the side of the follicle?
    a. Pseudofolliculitis barbae.   c. Tinea favosa.
    b. Pediculosis capitis.   d. Folliculitis barbae. _____

48. Folliculitis is the result of bacterial or viral infection and is characterized by _____.
    a. red papules or spots at the openings of the hair follicles
    b. dry, sulfur-yellow, cuplike crusts
    c. the inflammation or infection of one or more hair follicles
    d. itching, scales, and painful circular lesions _____

49. Dandruff is the result of _____.
    a. an active inflammatory process
    b. a fungus called malassezia
    c. an acute, deep-seated bacterial infection
    d. genetics _____

50. The term _____ is applied most frequently to a folliculitis barbae condition.
  a. razor bumps
  b. male pattern baldness
  c. barber's itch
  d. boil   ____

51. Which of the following is the result of an acute, deep-seated bacterial infection in the subcutaneous tissue?
  a. Carbuncle.   **c.** Razor bump.
  b. Boil.   **d.** Furuncle.   ____

52. Preparations that contain salicylic acid to break up impactions and kill bacteria are available for the prevention of _____.
  a. carbuncles   **c.** dandruff
  b. furuncles   **d.** ingrown hairs   ____

53. Do not proceed with _____ services if there are signs of irritation or abrasions.
  a. shaving   **c.** shampooing
  b. haircutting   **d.** chemical   ____

54. What type of hair is more susceptible to damage from chemical services?
  a. Coarse.   **c.** Medium.
  b. Fine.   **d.** Wiry.   ____

55. The number of hairs on the head varies with the _____ of the hair.
  a. elasticity   **c.** color
  b. coarseness   **d.** porosity   ____

56. What type of hair has a hard, glassy finish because the cuticle scales lie flat against the hair shaft?
  a. Wiry.   **c.** Fine.
  b. Coarse.   **d.** Medium.   ____

57. Hair that breaks easily or fails to return to its normal length _____.
  a. is over-porous   **c.** has low pH
  b. has low elasticity   **d.** is more alkaline   ____

58. Hair with a high porosity level is considered overly porous and is usually the result of _____.
   a. hormonal changes
   b. internal disorders
   c. poor nutrition
   d. previous over-processing ____

59. The sense of _____ is key to analyzing hair condition and texture.
   a. touch
   b. smell
   c. sight
   d. hearing ____

60. It is more difficult for hair lighteners, haircolors, waving solutions, and relaxing creams to penetrate what type of hair?
   a. Fine.
   b. Wiry.
   c. Coarse.
   d. Wavy. ____

61. The degree of hair porosity is directly related to the condition of _____.
   a. abnormal hair growth
   b. the cuticle layer of the hair
   c. the endocrine glands
   d. a client's scalp ____

62. Hair _____ refers to the degree of coarseness or fineness of individual hair strands.
   a. density
   b. porosity
   c. texture
   d. elasticity ____

63. Hair with low or poor elasticity is _____.
   a. brittle and breaks easily
   b. over-porous
   c. more resistant to penetration
   d. very rough to the touch ____

64. What would hair be considered if it feels smooth and the cuticle is compact?
   a. Over-porous.
   b. Porous.
   c. Over processed.
   d. Resistant. ____

65. Hair with normal elasticity will stretch and return to its original length without _____.
   a. shedding
   b. tangling
   c. breaking
   d. knotting ____

66. The average hair density is approximately how many strands per square inch?

    a. 5,000.   **c.** 1,300.

    b. 2,200.   **d.** 10,000.   ____

67. Hair with low or poor elasticity may be the result of _____.

    a. poor nutrition   **c.** hair product

    b. genetics   **d.** age   ____

11 TREATMENT OF THE HAIR AND SCALP

MULTIPLE CHOICE

1. Follow-up conditioning treatments after the shampooing help to _____.
   a. prevent and combat disorders
   b. stimulate muscles
   c. increase blood circulation
   d. keep hair in a healthy and manageable condition ____

2. Shampooing the hair before cutting ensures that you are working with _____.
   a. clean hair
   b. practice and experience
   c. your thumbs and fingers
   d. even pressure and continuous synchronized movements ____

3. Shampoos are _____.
   a. ointments
   b. oil-in-water emulsions
   c. creams
   d. water-in-oil emulsions ____

4. What is the pH range for hair conditioners?
   a. 2.0 to 4.5.
   b. 3.0 to 5.5.
   c. 4.5 to 7.5.
   d. 6.0 to 8.5. ____

5. Which of the following would be used to treat conditions requiring a medicinal product?
   a. Shampoos.
   b. Hair conditioners.
   c. Finishing rinse.
   d. Scalp conditioners. ____

6. _____ moisturize the hair and help to restore some of the oils and/or proteins.
   a. Scalp conditioners
   b. Permanents
   c. Hair conditioners
   d. Shampoos ____

7. Wet hair has a tendency to stick to what type of capes?
   a. Nylon.
   b. Vinyl.
   c. Synthetic material.
   d. Terry cloth. ____

8. What type of barbering service requires either a neck strip or a cloth towel placed under and then folded over the neckband of the cape?
   a. Mustache/beard trim.
   b. Shave.
   c. Chemical.
   d. Shampoo. ____

9. One important guideline that applies to all draping methods is to _____.
   a. always have a cloth towel under the cape
   b. ask the client to remove delicate clothing
   c. wash your hands
   d. turn the client's collar to the outside if applicable ____

10. If a _____ service precedes the haircut, replace the vinyl cape and towel with a nylon cape and neck strip.
    a. shampoo
    b. shave
    c. chemical
    d. mustache/beard trim ____

11. Which of the following is a basic consideration for performing a shampoo service?
    a. Proper shampoo selection.
    b. Proper scalp treatments.
    c. Proper hygienic practices.
    d. Proper body positioning of the barber. ____

12. The _____ shampoo bowl is a freestanding unit that allows the barber to stand in back of the client's head.
    a. inclined
    b. European-style
    c. reclined
    d. standard ____

13. What shampooing method would require the client to bend his head forward over the shampoo bowl or sink?
    a. Reclined.
    b. Scalp massage.
    c. Inclined.
    d. Draping. ____

14. Some wheelchairs can be positioned comfortably at the shampoo bowl, while others may require the client to use the _____ shampooing method.
    a. safety
    b. inclined
    c. special needs
    d. reclined ____

15. To prevent muscle aches, back strain, and fatigue, it is important that you maintain _____ at the shampoo bowl.
   a. good posture
   b. compliance with state barber laws
   c. barber rules and regulations
   d. proper positioning of the client   ____

16. Hot water can cause the scalp to _____.
   a. become more flexible
   b. reduce the lathering of shampoos
   c. become oily
   d. flake or become dry   ____

17. Which of the following is *not* a characteristic of hair that should be considered before choosing products?
   a. Condition.   **c.** Color.
   b. Texture.   **d.** Density.   ____

18. A common reason that a client might find fault with the shampoo service could be _____.
   a. extreme water temperatures
   b. wetting or soiling the draping
   c. insufficient scraping of the client's scalp
   d. extreme scalp massage   ____

19. What type of hair may require a humectant-rich moisturizing conditioner to increase manageability?
   a. Chemically treated.   **c.** Oily.
   b. Dry, coarse.   **d.** Fine, brittle.   ____

20. _____ conditioners can weigh down fine hair, leaving it flat or oily.
   a. Light leave-in   **c.** Cuticle-coating
   b. Scalp   **d.** Spray-on   ____

21. What type of massage manipulation movement uses the thumbs and/or fingertips to produce overlapping circular movements?
   a. Rotary movement.
   b. Back and forth movement.
   c. Sliding movement.
   d. Firm pressure movement.   ____

22. Massage manipulations should be _____.
    a. performed with unsynchronized movements
    b. performed with intensity
    c. performed once a week
    d. slow and rhythmic   ____

23. Where do massage manipulations performed during a
    shampoo or scalp treatment start?
    a. Hairline.   c. Top of the head.
    b. Nape of the neck.   d. Back of the head.   ____

24. Oily scalp and hair is most often caused by _____.
    a. the fungus malassezia
    b. overactive sebaceous glands
    c. inactivity of the oil glands
    d. poor blood circulation to the scalp   ____

25. Which of the following is effective in preparing the scalp for
    scalp massage manipulations and treatments?
    a. Hair tonic.   c. Scalp steam.
    b. Electric massager.   d. Hand massager.   ____

26. Scalp steamers, steam towels, vibrators, and scalp
    manipulations may all be used with _____.
    a. protein treatments
    b. leave-in conditioners
    c. gentle cleansing shampoos
    d. hair tonics   ____

27. Which of the following is the term used to describe abnormal
    hair loss?
    a. Pediculosis capitis.   c. Malassezia.
    b. Alopecia.   d. Dandruff.   ____

28. If abrasions or lesions are present, you should not
    recommend what type of service?
    a. Haircutting.
    b. Shampoo massage.
    c. Powder shampoo application.
    d. Scalp steam.   ____

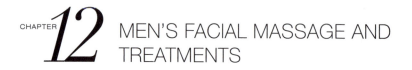

CHAPTER 12 MEN'S FACIAL MASSAGE AND TREATMENTS

MULTIPLE CHOICE

1. An example of an electric current modality is
   _____.
   - **a.** electric massager
   - **b.** light-emitting diode
   - **c.** galvanic
   - **d.** heat lamp   ____

2. _____ is an example of a heat modality.
   - **a.** Microcurrent
   - **b.** Low-level light therapy
   - **c.** Low-level laser therapy
   - **d.** Infrared device   ____

3. What muscle covers the back of the neck, allowing movement of the shoulders?
   - **a.** Platysma.
   - **b.** Trapezius.
   - **c.** Sternocleidomastoideus.
   - **d.** Triangularis.   ____

4. The broad muscle that covers the top of the skull is the _____ muscle.
   - **a.** Epicranius
   - **b.** Frontalis
   - **c.** Epicranial aponeurosis
   - **d.** Occipitalis   ____

5. Which of the following is an example of a chemical modality?
   - **a.** Galvanic.
   - **b.** Lasers.
   - **c.** Microdermabrasion.
   - **d.** Microcurrent.   ____

6. The muscles that coordinate opening and closing the mouth are the _____ muscles.
   - **a.** buccinator
   - **b.** mentalis
   - **c.** risorius
   - **d.** masseter   ____

7. Which of the following is the tendon that connects the occipitalis and frontalis?
   - **a.** Epicranius.
   - **b.** Epicranial aponeurosis.
   - **c.** Corrugator.
   - **d.** Procerus.   ____

8. What muscle is used when laughing?
   - **a.** Zygomaticus major.
   - **b.** Mentalis.
   - **c.** Orbicularis oris.
   - **d.** Triangularis.   ____

70

9. What muscle bends and rotates the head?
   a. Zygomaticus minor.
   b. Trapezius.
   c. Sternocleidomastoideus.
   d. Platysma.   ____

10. A hot towel is an example of what type of nerve response modality?
   a. Massage.   c. Heat.
   b. Moist heat.   d. Current.   ____

11. Heat and moist heat on the skin cause _____ .
   a. relaxation   c. stimulation
   b. contraction   d. constriction   ____

12. Which of the following is an example of an electric current modality?
   a. Laser.   c. High frequency.
   b. Infrared device.   d. Electric massager.   ____

13. What nerve is the chief sensory nerve of the face?
   a. Facial.   c. Seventh cranial.
   b. Eleventh cranial.   d. Fifth cranial.   ____

14. The motor nerve that controls motions of the neck muscles is the _____ nerve.
   a. seventh cranial   c. trifacial
   b. accessory   d. fifth cranial   ____

15. The fifth cranial nerve is also known as the _____ nerve.
   a. cervical   c. trigeminal
   b. accessory   d. facial   ____

16. What nerve branches supply the muscles and scalp at the back of the head and neck?
   a. Trigeminal.   c. Accessory.
   b. Eleventh cranial.   d. Spinal.   ____

17. How many pairs of cranial nerves are connected to a part of the brain surface?
   a. 6.   c. 18.
   b. 12.   d. 24.   ____

18. _____ are vessels that transport oxygenated blood from the heart to all parts of the body.
- **a.** Venules
- **b.** Arteries
- **c.** Capillaries
- **d.** Veins

_____

19. What arteries are the main sources of blood supply to the head, face, and neck?
- **a.** Superficial temporals.
- **b.** External maxillaries.
- **c.** Common carotids.
- **d.** Posterior auriculars.

_____

20. Which of the following transport deoxygenated blood from various parts of the body to the heart?
- **a.** Veins.
- **b.** Arteries.
- **c.** Nerves.
- **d.** Lymph.

_____

21. _____ is a stroking movement.
- **a.** Percussion
- **b.** Pétrissage
- **c.** Effleurage
- **d.** Friction

_____

22. Which of the following is the most stimulating form of massage?
- **a.** Pétrissage.
- **b.** Percussion.
- **c.** Friction.
- **d.** Effleurage.

_____

23. What type of massage movements are the gentlest form of tapotement?
- **a.** Tapping.
- **b.** Hacking.
- **c.** Kneading.
- **d.** Stroking.

_____

24. What massage movement exerts an invigorating effect on the area being massaged?
- **a.** Effleurage.
- **b.** Percussion.
- **c.** Tapotement.
- **d.** Pétrissage.

_____

25. Which of the following should be used sparingly and not exceed a few seconds' duration on any one area?
- **a.** Tapotement.
- **b.** Percussion.
- **c.** Vibration.
- **d.** Friction.

_____

26. _____ should only be used on the back and shoulders.
- **a.** Rubbing
- **b.** Hacking
- **c.** Slapping
- **d.** Tapping

_____

27. What massage manipulation has proven to be beneficial to the circulation and glandular activity of the skin?
- **a.** Friction.
- **b.** Percussion.
- **c.** Tapotement.
- **d.** Vibration.

_____

28. In what type of movements are the lower points to midpoints of the fingers used to strike the skin lightly and rapidly?
a. Tapping.
c. Chopping.
b. Hacking.
d. Slapping.
____

29. What type of massage movement stimulates the nerves to tone the muscles?
a. Effleurage.
c. Percussion.
b. Pétrissage.
d. Friction.
____

30. Deep vibration with a mechanical vibrator or massager can _____.
a. have a relaxing effect
b. impart a healthy glow to the part being massaged
c. improve glandular activity
d. stimulate blood circulation
____

31. When electrical stimulation is applied to the nerve through electrodes, the muscle responds by _____.
a. contracting
c. relaxing
b. expanding
d. stretching
____

32. A _____ point is a point on the skin where nerves that control the underlying muscle are located.
a. functional
c. localized
b. motor
d. trigger
____

33. Which of the following is a beneficial result that may be obtained by proper massage?
a. Muscle fiber is reduced.
b. Nerves are stimulated.
c. Circulation of blood is increased.
d. Circulation of blood is decreased.
____

34. A trigger point exhibits hypersensitivity to _____.
a. chemicals
c. light rays
b. moist heat
d. electrical stimulation
____

35. Where is the immediate effect of massage first noticed?
a. In the nerves.
c. In the muscles.
b. Blood circulation.
d. On the skin.
____

36. A beneficial result obtained by proper massage is that
_____ .
   a. circulation of blood is decreased
   b. muscle fiber is soothed
   c. fat cells are reduced
   d. nerves are strengthened ____

37. The _____ of a muscle is the attachment point to a
movable bone.
   a. trigger   **c.** base
   b. insertion   **d.** origin ____

38. Massage should never be recommended or employed when
_____ is present.
   a. high blood pressure   **c.** a hypertrophy
   b. low blood pressure   **d.** a keloid ____

39. Which of the following helps to soften follicle accumulation?
   a. Galvanic machine.   **c.** Steam.
   b. High-frequency current.   **d.** Brushing. ____

40. The primary actions of high-frequency current are thermal
and _____ .
   a. systematic   **c.** therapeutic
   b. tonic   **d.** antiseptic ____

41. Overexposure to _____ can destroy skin tissue.
   a. alkaline-pH products   **c.** ultraviolet rays
   b. microcrystals   **d.** astringent solutions ____

42. Which of the following heats and relaxes the skin without
increasing overall body temperature?
   a. Ultraviolet rays.   **c.** Microcurrents.
   b. Infrared rays.   **d.** Galvanic currents. ____

43. _____ is the use of the positive pole (anode) to
introduce an acid-pH product into the skin.
   a. Cataphoresis   **c.** Anaphoresis
   b. Desincrustation   **d.** Iontophoresis ____

44. To perform desincrustation, a(n) _____ solution is
applied to the skin's surface.
   a. alkaline-pH
   b. astringent
   c. ion-containing water-soluble
   d. acid-based ____

45. Which of the following is a form of mechanical exfoliation?
   a. Direct surface application.　　**c.** Brushing.
   b. Desincrustation.　　**d.** Steaming.　　____

46. _____ produces fast, visible results and can be used to treat surface wrinkles and aging skin.
   a. Light therapy　　**c.** Anaphoresis
   b. Microdermabrasion　　**d.** Cataphoresis　　____

47. What is a type of galvanic treatment that uses a very low level of electrical current for applications in skin care?
   a. Microcurrent.　　**c.** Iontophoresis.
   b. Microdermabrasion.　　**d.** Desincrustation.　　____

48. The high-frequency machine can benefit the client's skin by _____.
   a. deoxygenating the skin
   b. decreasing blood circulation
   c. decreasing glandular activity
   d. increasing cell metabolism　　____

49. A negative electrode is known as a(n) _____.
   a. anode　　**c.** cathode
   b. high-frequency current　　**d.** wavelength　　____

50. Ultraviolet lamps may be used to treat _____.
   a. nerve disorders　　**c.** dandruff
   b. wrinkles　　**d.** aging skin　　____

51. _____ is (are) used to produce chemical and ionic reactions in the skin.
   a. Tesla current　　**c.** Galvanic current
   b. High-frequency current　　**d.** Ultraviolet rays　　____

52. Which of the following should never be performed on skin that has been treated with Retin-A®?
   a. Light therapy.　　**c.** Desincrustation.
   b. Cataphoresis.　　**d.** Brushing.　　____

53. What type of skin treatment can assist the body in producing vitamin D?
   a. Ultraviolet lamps.　　**c.** Microdermabrasion.
   b. Infrared rays.　　**d.** Microcurrents.　　____

54. Which of the following relieves pain in sore muscles?
   a. Desincrustation.　　**c.** High-frequency current.
   b. Infrared rays.　　**d.** Ultraviolet rays.　　____

55. For general facial or scalp treatments, no more than 5 minutes should be allowed for _____.
   a. brushing
   b. facial steaming
   c. high-frequency current
   d. hot towels ____

56. With oily skin, the follicle size is _____.
   a. deeper
   b. smaller
   c. rounder
   d. larger ____

57. What type of products work best for combination skin types?
   a. Alcohol-based.
   b. Oil-based.
   c. Water-based.
   d. Water-oil-based. ____

58. Cleansing creams are used to _____.
   a. soften the skin
   b. dissolve dirt and makeup
   c. rebalance the pH of the skin
   d. prevent moisture from evaporating ____

59. Which of the following can work as an astringent?
   a. Witch hazel.
   b. Humectants.
   c. Emollients.
   d. Paraffin wax. ____

60. What type of skin is caused by an insufficient flow of sebum from the sebaceous glands?
   a. Normal.
   b. Oily.
   c. Combination.
   d. Dry. ____

61. Acne is a disorder of the _____ glands.
   a. seborrheic
   b. thyroid
   c. sebaceous
   d. endocrine ____

62. What type of mask uses hydrators and soothing ingredients to add moisture to sensitive or dehydrated skin?
   a. Cream.
   b. Paraffin wax.
   c. Clay.
   d. Gel. ____

63. _____ masks are used to stimulate circulation and temporarily contract the skin pores.
   a. Paraffin wax
   b. Clay
   c. Gel
   d. Cream ____

64. Which of the following is an example of a chemical exfoliant?
   a. Enzyme peel.   **c.** Granular scrub.
   b. Emollient.   **d.** Astringent.   ____

65. Toners are designed to _____.
   a. draw impurities out of pores
   b. add moisture to the skin surface
   c. tighten the skin
   d. remove dead cells from the skin surface   ____

66. The T-zone is the section of the face that incorporates the forehead, nose, and _____.
   a. upper neck area   **c.** cheekbones
   b. chin   **d.** lips   ____

67. Proper _____ and a water-based hydrator help keep oily skin clean and balanced.
   a. exfoliation   **c.** vibration
   b. massage   **d.** circulation   ____

68. Masks help to _____.
   a. loosen the skin
   b. dissolve dead-cell buildup on the skin surface
   c. soften the skin
   d. draw impurities out of pores   ____

69. Astringents may contain up to _____ percent alcohol.
   a. 15   **c.** 35
   b. 20   **d.** 50   ____

70. High-quality masks and packs should feel comfortable while producing slight _____ sensations.
   a. scratching   **c.** tingling
   b. soothing   **d.** relaxing   ____

71. What type of mask employs the pack application method?
   a. Cream.   **c.** Clay.
   b. Paraffin wax.   **d.** Gel.   ____

72. A mask is a(n) _____ product providing complete closure to the environment on top of the skin.
   a. setting   **c.** alkaline-pH
   b. water-based   **d.** acid-pH   ____

73. Dry skin facials can be supplemented with _____ rays.
    a. UVB   **c.** infrared
    b. UVA   **d.** UVC   ____

74. What type of treatment helps maintain the health of facial skin through correct cleansing, toning, and massage?
    a. Light therapy.   **c.** Microdermabrasion.
    b. Corrective.   **d.** Preservative.   ____

75. Alipidic skin is also known as _____ skin.
    a. dry   **c.** normal
    b. oily   **d.** combination   ____

76. The sebaceous material in a follicle darkens when it is exposed to _____ and forms a blackhead.
    a. cleansers   **c.** oxygen
    b. oil   **d.** water   ____

CHAPTER 13 SHAVING AND FACIAL-HAIR DESIGN

MULTIPLE CHOICE

1. Which of the following will you not perform immediately after a shave?
   a. Second-time-over shave.
   b. Deep cleansing facial.
   c. Applying fresheners or toners.
   d. Applying a warm towel. ____

2. The application of _____ is a standard procedure in preparing the beard for shaving.
   a. toners
   b. fresheners
   c. hot towels
   d. astringents ____

3. Do not proceed with the shave service if the client has

   _____.
   a. pustules
   b. whorl growth patterns
   c. chapped skin
   d. a keloid condition ____

4. What determines hairline shapes?
   a. Skin type.
   b. Facial-hair design.
   c. Hair texture.
   d. Growth patterns. ____

5. _____ are often the result of improper hair removal by a razor, tweezers, or trimmer.
   a. Pustules
   b. Skin infections
   c. Ingrown hairs
   d. Whorls ____

6. Do not use hot towels on skin that is _____.
   a. tanned
   b. chapped
   c. wrinkled
   d. freckled ____

7. Be careful when shaving sensitive areas such as

   _____.
   a. around the Adam's apple
   b. on the cheekbones
   c. upper part of the neck
   d. on top of the lip ____

8. When a client wears a mustache, trim and shape it
_____ the shave service.

   a. closer than   **c.** during

   b. after   **d.** prior to   ____

9. Ingrown hairs are also known as _____ .

   a. pustules   **c.** pseudofolliculitis

   b. folliculitis   **d.** a keloid condition   ____

10. Which of the following is a reason a client may find fault with
a shave procedure?

   a. Warm fingers.   **c.** Sharp razors.

   b. Heavy touch.   **d.** Soft overhead lights.   ____

11. There are 14 shaving areas of the face to be shaved during
the _____ part of the service.

   a. close shave   **c.** first-time-over

   b. second-time-over   **d.** once-over shave   ____

12. The 14 shaving areas of the face are shaved _____
and sequentially from one section to another.

   a. quickly   **c.** diagonally

   b. repeatedly   **d.** systematically   ____

13. During the first-time-over part of the service, you would
shave _____ in each of the 14 areas of the face.

   a. with the grain   **c.** across the grain

   b. against the grain   **d.** in a circular manner   ____

14. The shaving movement from the angle of mouth toward
point of chin would be which of the following?

   a. Freehand and down.

   b. Backhand and down.

   c. Reverse freehand and up.

   d. Freehand and across.   ____

15. The shaving movement from beneath the lower lip would be
_____ .

   a. backhand and down

   b. freehand and down

   c. reverse freehand and up

   d. backhand and down   ____

16. What type of strokes do you use around the mouth, over the
ears, and in other tight areas?

   a. Faster.   **c.** Medium.

   b. Shorter.   **d.** Longer.   ____

17. Lathering with a shaving cream or gel _____.
    a. softens the hair cuticle
    b. provides lubrication by stimulating oil glands
    c. relaxes the client
    d. cleanses the skin   ____

18. Stretching the skin too tightly will cause _____.
    a. nicks   **c.** irritation
    b. cuts   **d.** ingrown hairs   ____

19. What type of shaving is the practice of shaving the beard against the grain during the second-time-over phase of the shave?
    a. Close.   **c.** Outline.
    b. Once-over shave.   **d.** Complete.   ____

20. What type of shave should result in a smooth face without being a close shave?
    a. Outline.   **c.** Second-time-over.
    b. First-time-over.   **d.** Once-over shave.   ____

21. For a man who has an extra-large mouth, what type of mustache would be complimentary?
    a. Heavier-looking.   **c.** Semi-square.
    b. Pyramid-shaped.   **d.** Medium to large.   ____

22. Beards can be used to _____ the appearance of facial features.
    a. dominant   **c.** balance
    b. minimize   **d.** perfect   ____

23. You should angle the razor how many degrees relative to the skin surface?
    a. 10 degrees.   **c.** 45 degrees.
    b. 30 degrees.   **d.** 90 degrees.   ____

24. The correct angle of cutting with a razor is called the _____ stroke.
    a. cutting   **c.** gliding
    b. freehand   **d.** proper   ____

25. Which of the following refers to the way the razor is held in the barber's hand to perform a stroke movement?
    a. Angle.   **c.** Position.
    b. Grain.   **d.** Procedure.   ____

26. You would apply light facial cream or moisturizing lotion with what type of movement?
    a. Pétrissage massage.
    c. Sliding.
    b. Forward gliding.
    d. Effleurage massage.   ____

27. Right-handed barbers stand at the client's _____ .
    a. right side
    c. left side
    b. back
    d. front   ____

28. Which of the following is an antihemorrhagic?
    a. Alcohol.
    b. Astringent.
    c. Styptic powder.
    d. pH-balanced fresheners or toners.   ____

29. What razor position and stroke is *not* used in facial shaving?
    a. Freehand.
    c. Backhand.
    b. Reverse backhand.
    d. Reverse freehand.   ____

30. When performing a shave service, you would use the _____ to stretch the skin with the proper amount of pressure.
    a. cushions of the fingertips
    c. palms
    b. thumbs
    d. little fingers   ____

31. The reverse-backhand stroke is only used during a _____ shave.
    a. once-over
    c. first-time-over
    b. neck
    d. second-time-over   ____

32. Preparation includes which of the following?
    a. Light powder dusting.
    b. Toning.
    c. Draping the client.
    d. Massaging moisturizer into the skin.   ____

33. Steaming helps to _____ .
    a. hold the hair in an upright position
    b. cleanse the skin
    c. create a smooth surface for the razor
    d. provide lubrication by stimulating oil glands   ____

34. What type of skin allows the beard hair to be cut more easily?
    a. Taut.
    c. Tight.
    b. Loose.
    d. Dry.   ____

35. Which of the following shaves should ensure a complete and even shave with a single lathering?
    a. First-time-over.
    b. Close.
    c. Once-over shave.
    d. Second-time-over.   ____

36. Be sure to check the hairline and neck areas for _____ before beginning the neck shave.
    a. rough or uneven spots
    b. hypertrophies
    c. taut skin
    d. ingrown hairs   ____

37. _____ cutting is most successful on beards with even density and texture.
    a. Razor cutting
    b. Shear-over-comb
    c. Outliner-over-comb
    d. Even-all-over clipper   ____

38. Following the first-time-over shave, the barber checks the client's skin for any _____ .
    a. cuts
    b. hypertrophies
    c. rough or uneven spots
    d. nicks   ____

39. Finishing a shave would include which of the following?
    a. Steaming the face.
    b. Massaging moisturizer into the skin.
    c. Stretching the skin.
    d. Lathering the face with cream or gel.   ____

40. When performing a shave service, you should keep the nondominant thumb and fingertips dry for _____ purposes.
    a. stretching
    b. stroking
    c. positioning
    d. finishing   ____

41. Do not stop short or shave over an area _____ .
    a. systematically
    b. gently
    c. repeatedly
    d. sequentially   ____

42. Keep your fingers _____ to stretch or hold the skin firmly during the shave.
    a. powdered
    b. dry
    c. gloved
    d. moist   ____

43. When performing a shave, you would use a light touch and what type of motion that leads with the point of the blade?
    a. Very fast.
    b. Very slow.
    c. Sliding.
    d. Forward gliding.   ____

44. Where should you discard used blades?
  a. Trash basket. **c.** Sharps container.
  b. Plastic garbage bag. **d.** Closed receptacle. ____

45. Keep the skin _____ while shaving.
  a. hot **c.** dry
  b. moist **d.** cold ____

46. Treat small cuts or nicks using standard precautions and _____ procedures.
  a. exposure incident **c.** disinfectant
  b. first aid **d.** safety ____

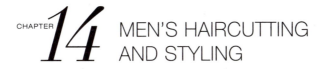

CHAPTER **14** MEN'S HAIRCUTTING AND STYLING

MULTIPLE CHOICE

1. What might you discover during the client consultation that may prohibit moving forward with the service?
   a. Undesirable outcomes.
   b. Scalp conditions.
   c. Lifestyle choices.
   d. Hair conditions. ____

2. What is the average rate of hair growth per month?
   a. ¼ inch.   **c.** 1 inch.
   b. 1½ inches.   **d.** ½ inch. ____

3. Asking questions of the client during the consultation helps you properly complete the process of _____.
   a. informing   **c.** envisioning
   b. communicating   **d.** analyzing ____

4. What facial shape has over-wide cheekbones and a narrow jaw line?
   a. Inverted triangular.   **c.** Pear-shaped.
   b. Oval.   **d.** Diamond. ____

5. With what facial shape would you direct bangs off the face and into the sides to broaden the appearance of the forehead?
   a. Inverted triangular.   **c.** Diamond.
   b. Square.   **d.** Round. ____

6. With the _____ facial shape, layered bangs brushed to the sides over the temples can give the illusion of a shorter facial shape.
   a. oval   **c.** diamond
   b. oblong   **d.** pear-shaped ____

7. Which of the following facial shapes is recognized as the ideal shape?
   a. Oblong.   **c.** Round.
   b. Square.   **d.** Oval. ____

8. What type of profile has a prominent forehead and chin?
- **a.** Concave.
- **b.** Straight.
- **c.** Convex.
- **d.** Angular.

____

9. What facial profile can appear more balanced by arranging the hair over the forehead and by adding a mustache and a close-cut beard?
- **a.** Straight.
- **b.** Concave.
- **c.** Angular.
- **d.** Convex.

____

10. With what facial profile would you use a close hair arrangement at the forehead to minimize the bulge of the forehead?
- **a.** Angular.
- **b.** Convex.
- **c.** Straight.
- **d.** Concave.

____

11. A long neck can appear shorter if the hair is left fuller or longer at the _____ .
- **a.** ears
- **b.** chin
- **c.** nape
- **d.** shoulder

____

12. For what facial shape would you create some height on the top to lengthen the look of the face?
- **a.** Diamond.
- **b.** Pear-shaped.
- **c.** Square.
- **d.** Round.

____

13. What type of beard would help to fill out a narrow jaw?
- **a.** Full.
- **b.** Close-cut.
- **c.** Rounded.
- **d.** Square.

____

14. The _____ is the widest section of the head, starting at the temples and ending just below the crown.
- **a.** apex
- **b.** parietal ridge
- **c.** occipital bone
- **d.** four corners

____

15. The parietal ridge is also known as the _____ .
- **a.** horseshoe
- **b.** projection
- **c.** guideline
- **d.** apex

____

16. Which of the following is used to establish proportionate design lines and contours?
- **a.** Guides.
- **b.** Reference points.
- **c.** Partings.
- **d.** Cutting lines.

____

17. What type of hairstyle is tapered slightly higher to above the occipital?
   a. Fade.
   b. Longer.
   c. Medium-length.
   d. Semi-short. ____

18. The primary tapering areas of a cut are determined by the _____ .
   a. natural part
   b. design line
   c. style
   d. client's preference ____

19. Medium-length styles do not have a _____ appearance.
   a. scalped
   b. uniform
   c. finished
   d. full ____

20. Vertical cutting lines _____.
   a. create sloped lines within a haircut
   b. build weight
   c. remove weight within the cut
   d. create a stacked, layered effect ____

21. _____ refers to the quality of a form's surface.
   a. Weight line
   b. Design texture
   c. Proportion
   d. Trough ____

22. What type of cutting line is used to create a one-length look and low elevation or blunt haircut designs?
   a. Curved.
   b. Diagonal.
   c. Vertical.
   d. Horizontal. ____

23. Curved lines _____.
   a. soften a design
   b. create a one-length look
   c. create sloped lines
   d. remove weight within the cut ____

24. Which of the following is an important design element when discussing balance?
   a. Hair texture.
   b. Hair porosity.
   c. Hair density.
   d. Hair color. ____

25. A(n) _____ is a series of connected dots that result in a continuous mark.
   a. outline
   b. shape
   c. form
   d. line ____

26. _____ help to create strong, consistent foundations in haircutting.
    a. Angles
    b. Lines
    c. Forms
    d. Elevations   ____

27. Cutting _____ is cutting the hair in the same direction in which it grows.
    a. across the grain
    b. with the grain
    c. against the grain
    d. with a circular motion   ____

28. _____ cutting creates crisp, clean lines at the hairline on shorter hairstyles.
    a. 180-degree elevation
    b. 45-degree elevation
    c. 0-elevation
    d. 90-degree elevation   ____

29. The _____ is the outer perimeter line of the haircut.
    a. guideline
    b. parting
    c. cutting line
    d. design line   ____

30. A stationary guide is used for _____ .
    a. achieving overall one-length-looking designs at the perimeter
    b. texturizing or removing bulk in the hair
    c. cutting tightly curled hair
    d. elevating the hair beyond zero elevation   ____

31. _____ is the angle or degree at which a section of hair is held from the head for cutting, relative from where it grows.
    a. Position
    b. Direction
    c. Elevation
    d. Transition   ____

32. What amount of tension is used on straight hair to create precise lines?
    a. Moderate.
    b. Maximum.
    c. Minimum.
    d. Medium.   ____

33. Most men's haircuts require some form of _____ .
    a. layering
    b. texturing
    c. thinning
    d. tapering   ____

34. A _____ line refers to the heaviest perimeter area of a 0-elevation or 45-degree cut.
    a. weight
    b. cutting
    c. vertical
    d. horizontal   ____

35. Which of the following creates a length increase in the design?
   a. Texturizing.
   c. Layering.
   b. Overdirection.
   d. Tapering.   ____

36. _____ is frequently used in men's haircutting to cut and blend layers in the top, crown, and horseshoe areas.
   a. Cutting below the fingers
   b. Shear-over-comb
   c. Cutting palm-to-palm
   d. Cutting above the fingers   ____

37. What technique is most often used to create design lines at the perimeter of the haircut?
   a. Cutting palm-to-palm.
   b. Cutting above the fingers.
   c. Cutting below the fingers.
   d. Freehand shear cutting.   ____

38. Which of the following is used to thin out or customize difficult areas caused by hollows, wrinkles, whorls, or creases in the scalp?
   a. Shear-point tapering.
   b. Freehand shear cutting.
   c. Clipper-over-comb.
   d. Freehand clipper cutting.   ____

39. What cutting techniques are used for longer, tightly curled hair lengths that require more sculpting?
   a. Clipper-over-comb.
   c. Razor.
   b. Freehand clipper.
   d. Freehand shear.   ____

40. What cutting technique is also known as freehand slicing?
   a. Razor-over-comb.
   b. Freehand clipper.
   c. Razor rotation.
   d. Fingers-and-razor.   ____

41. In _____ the razor is held almost flat against the surface of the hair.
   a. light taper-blending
   b. terminal blending
   c. thinning
   d. heavier taper-blending   ____

42. With what type of hair do you use a light stroke of the razor with very little pressure?
    a. Coarse.
    b. Fine.
    c. Thick.
    d. Medium-textured. _____

43. For razor cutting, the hair must be clean and _____ for best results.
    a. moisturized
    b. wet
    c. damp
    d. dry _____

44. The shear-over-comb technique is used to cut the ends of the hair and is used in _____ .
    a. trimming
    b. layering
    c. texturing
    d. tapering _____

45. Which of the following may cause injury to your fingers?
    a. Shear blades resting near to the fingers.
    b. Shear blades resting flat to the fingers.
    c. Angling the shear blades.
    d. Shear blades resting flush to the fingers. _____

46. For which of the following cuts should the top of the crest area look squared off when viewed from the front?
    a. Precision cut.
    b. Flat top.
    c. Fade style.
    d. Taper cut. _____

47. The _____ is a medium to long taper cut with a long top section.
    a. classic pompadour
    b. butch cut
    c. quo vadis
    d. classic Caesar _____

48. Which of the following cuts is a variation of the crew cut?
    a. Precision cut.
    b. Princeton cut.
    c. Flat top.
    d. Brush cut. _____

49. The _____ is cut with shears to create short, uniform layers.
    a. flat top
    b. crew cut
    c. classic Caesar
    d. pompadour fade _____

50. Which of the following is a variation of the taper cut?
    a. Butch cut.
    b. Businessman's cut.
    c. Brush cut.
    d. Quo vadis cut. _____

51. What is the most popular technique for eyebrow trimming?
    a. Clipper-over-comb.
    b. Cutting below the fingers.
    c. Razor cutting.
    d. Shear-over-comb. _____

52. What is often included as part of the outline shave in many African American styles?
a. Nostril hair trimming.
b. Ear hair trimming.
c. Front hairline shaving.
d. Eyebrow trimming.   ____

53. When shaving the head, the hair and scalp are prepared with _____ and lather.
a. hot towels
b. moisturizers
c. non-petroleum-based oils
d. a massage   ____

54. Trimming excess hair in or around the ears is performed with _____ .
a. a straight razor   c. an electric razor
b. an outliner   d. shears   ____

55. Before shaving the head, thoroughly analyze the scalp to identify _____ .
a. the sections of the head
b. hair density
c. hypertrophies
d. hair growth patterns   ____

56. Which of the following was popular for both men and women during the 1920s and 1930s?
a. Braiding.   c. Diffused drying.
b. Finger waving.   d. Scrunch styling.   ____

57. _____ require(s) working close to the scalp across the curves of the head.
a. Cornrows   c. Scrunch styling
b. Finger waving   d. Blow waving   ____

58. What type of drying occurs when the hair is combed into place or arranged with the fingers and allowed to dry in place?
a. Stylized blow.   c. Freeform.
b. Diffused.   d. Natural.   ____

59. _____ are created from natural-textured hair that is intertwined together to form a single network of hair.
a. Braids   c. Locks
b. Cornrows   d. Twists   ____

60. Once the hair locks into compacted coils, it may be shampooed regularly and managed with a _____.
- **a.** non-petroleum-based oil
- **c.** pomade
- **b.** moisturizer
- **d.** styling gel

_____

61. Stylized blowdrying creates _____.
- **a.** a more finished appearance
- **b.** a natural wave pattern
- **c.** extra volume
- **d.** an even contour throughout the hair

_____

62. _____ is a wet styling technique that shapes and directs the hair into an S pattern.
- **a.** Double twisting
- **c.** Finger waving
- **b.** Scrunch styling
- **d.** Coiling

_____

63. Keep the air and the hair moving when blowdry styling to prevent _____.
- **a.** physical changes in the hair
- **b.** burning the client's scalp
- **c.** temporary straightening
- **d.** scrunching the hair

_____

64. The use of a razor with a _____ is recommended for the beginner.
- **a.** tempered blade
- **c.** changeable blade
- **b.** dull blade
- **d.** safety guard

_____

65. You should use what type of movement when raising or lowering chairs and seat backs?
- **a.** Brisk.
- **c.** Fast.
- **b.** Slow.
- **d.** Smooth.

_____

66. Safety and protection of the client's _____ should be the first consideration when using eyebrow-trimming techniques.
- **a.** temples
- **c.** eyes
- **b.** forehead
- **d.** skin

_____

67. Avoid applying _____ in one place on the head for too long.
- **a.** dryer heat
- **c.** lather
- **b.** pressure
- **d.** witch hazel

_____

68. You should keep a razor _____ whenever not in use.
- **a.** empty of a blade
- **c.** in a sharps container
- **b.** closed
- **d.** open

_____

15 MEN'S HAIR REPLACEMENT

MULTIPLE CHOICE

1. During the eighteenth century, what term was used to describe the front section of hair?
   - **a.** Queue.
   - **b.** Toupee.
   - **c.** Periwig.
   - **d.** Club. _____

2. Some men choose to cover their thinning or bald areas because they feel it makes them look _____ .
   - **a.** younger
   - **b.** slimmer
   - **c.** fashionable
   - **d.** successful _____

3. When discussing hair replacement with your client, be sure to take a very personal and _____ approach.
   - **a.** slow
   - **b.** hard-sell
   - **c.** private
   - **d.** technical _____

4. Take the time during the consultation to explain the finer points of hair restoration, _____ , bonding methods, and different hair solutions.
   - **a.** styling
   - **b.** upkeep
   - **c.** storage
   - **d.** transport _____

5. Which of the following is the best evidence of pleased and satisfied clients?
   - **a.** Personal referrals.
   - **b.** Network fan page.
   - **c.** Social media marketing.
   - **d.** Client coupons. _____

6. The more natural looking the _____ of the hair, the less obvious the hair solution will appear.
   - **a.** density
   - **b.** texture
   - **c.** wave
   - **d.** color _____

7. What type of advertising can be inexpensive and profitable?
   - **a.** Radio.
   - **b.** Television.
   - **c.** Newspaper.
   - **d.** Billboard. _____

8. _____ hair can last a lifetime if the service is performed properly.

  a. Cover-up
  b. Transplanted
  c. Synthetic
  d. Cell regenerated _____

9. What topical medication for hair replacement has potential side effects that include weight gain and loss of sexual function?

  a. Finasteride.
  b. Rogaine.
  c. Minoxidil.
  d. Loniten. _____

10. Which of the following services can be offered in the barbershop?

  a. Flap surgery.
  b. Scalp reduction.
  c. Hair transplantation.
  d. Low-light laser therapy. _____

11. An advantage of human hair is that _____.

  a. it can be cleaned with cleaner solutions
  b. it does not oxidize
  c. it has the ability to tolerate chemical processes
  d. it does not lose its style _____

12. What type of hair product is often used in the manufacture of theatrical or fashion wigs?

  a. Chemically treated.
  b. Mixed.
  c. Human.
  d. Synthetic. _____

13. _____ hair has become the most popular choice when it comes to hair replacement.

  a. Human
  b. Mixed
  c. Synthetic
  d. Chemically treated _____

14. _____ refers to the way the hair is attached to the base of the hair solution.

  a. Fitting
  b. Looping
  c. Root-turning
  d. Knotting _____

15. A template or _____ analysis should be done prior to fitting any hair solution.

  a. contour
  b. custom
  c. consultation
  d. construction _____

16. Which of the following can be used as samples to show prospective hair replacement clients what a replacement system might look like?
  a. Window displays.
  b. Your own personal hair solution.
  c. Stock systems.
  d. Custom systems. _____

17. Which of the following supplies needed for hair solutions are not standard barbershop items?
  a. Small brushes.   **c.** Thinning shears.
  b. Adhesives.   **d.** Roller picks. _____

18. What type of hair solution is recommended when the hair is worn in an off-the-face style?
  a. Cover-up.   **c.** Partial lace fill-in.
  b. Full head bonding.   **d.** Lace-front. _____

19. Ready-to-wear wigs are usually made of _____ .
  a. a synthetic fiber   **c.** angora
  b. yak hair   **d.** wool _____

20. _____ is the process of attaching a hair replacement system to the head with an adhesive bonding agent.
  a. Lace-front   **c.** Partial lace fill-in
  b. Full head bonding   **d.** Partial hair solution _____

21. Synthetic hair solutions should always be cleaned with _____ .
  a. hot water   **c.** cold water
  b. re-conditioners   **d.** a solvent _____

22. Re-conditioning treatments should be given to prevent _____ of the hair.
  a. yellowing   **c.** dryness or brittleness
  b. fading   **d.** matting _____

23. You should brush and comb hair solutions with a(n) _____ movement.
  a. upward   **c.** brisk
  b. downward   **d.** diagonal _____

24. Which of the following is accomplished by using roller picks to support the rod above the base of the hair system?
    a. Knotting.
    b. Looping.
    c. Floating.
    d. Root-turning.   ____

25. Use _____ to blend the ends of the replacement with the client's natural hair.
    a. clippers
    b. trimmers
    c. a razor
    d. thinning shears   ____

26. After cutting and blending a full head bonded replacement system, allow _____ before shampooing.
    a. 12 hours
    b. 24 to 48 hours
    c. 5 days
    d. 1 week   ____

27. Taper gradually using a _____ method so the replacement system will be undetectable when blended with the client's natural hair.
    a. fingers-and-shear
    b. clipper-over-comb
    c. slide cutting
    d. thinning   ____

16 WOMEN'S HAIRCUTTING AND STYLING

MULTIPLE CHOICE

1. In women's haircutting, the lines along the hairline are usually _____ .
   - **a.** softer
   - **b.** shorter
   - **c.** more textured
   - **d.** more blunt

   _____

2. When cutting women's hair, take consistent, clean _____ to produce precise results.
   - **a.** layers
   - **b.** partings
   - **c.** razor cuts
   - **d.** elevations

   _____

3. In which of the following cuts do all the hair strands end at one level to form a heavy weight line at the perimeter?
   - **a.** Graduated.
   - **b.** Long-layered.
   - **c.** Blunt.
   - **d.** Uniform-layered.

   _____

4. The most common elevation for a graduated cut is _____ .
   - **a.** 0 degrees
   - **b.** 45 degrees
   - **c.** 90 degrees
   - **d.** 180 degrees

   _____

5. When finished, which cut will look soft and textured and conform to the head shape without weight lines or corners?
   - **a.** Blunt.
   - **b.** Uniform-layered.
   - **c.** Graduated.
   - **d.** Long-layered.

   _____

6. Which of the following cuts consists of increased layering achieved by cutting hair at a 180-degree elevation?
   - **a.** Uniform-layered.
   - **b.** Blunt.
   - **c.** Long-layered.
   - **d.** Graduated.

   _____

7. Thick, coarse curly hair types are easier to cut with the _____ .
   - **a.** clippers
   - **b.** shears
   - **c.** scissors
   - **d.** razor

   _____

8. Curly hair tends to graduate naturally due to the curl pattern
   and _____.
   a. mobility   c. elasticity
   b. density   d. texture   ____

9. Which of the following is the process of thinning the hair to
   graduated lengths with the shears?
   a. Texturing.   c. Carving.
   b. Slicing.   d. Slithering.   ____

10. _____ is performed at the ends of the hair using the
    tips of the shears at a steep shear angle in relation to the
    hair parting.
    a. Carving.   c. Notching
    b. Point cutting   d. Slicing   ____

11. What haircutting technique blends short and long lengths
    along a perimeter design line or interior section?
    a. Overdirection.   c. Texturizing.
    b. Razor cutting.   d. Notching.   ____

12. _____ set a pattern in the hair that will form the basis
    for a hairstyle.
    a. Curling irons   c. Rollers
    b. Hair wraps   d. Pin curls   ____

13. What part of the curl is the hair between the scalp and the
    first arc of the circle?
    a. Barrel.   c. Base.
    b. Foundation.   d. Stem.   ____

14. _____ is the process of shaping and directing the hair
    into an S-shaped pattern through the use of fingers, comb,
    and setting lotion.
    a. Thermal styling   c. Hair wrapping
    b. Finger waving   d. Hair molding   ____

15. Thermal waving is performed with _____.
    a. heated pressing combs   c. Marcel irons
    b. blowdryers   d. flat irons   ____

16. For a blunt cut, what should you *not* use when blowdrying,
    as it creates a bend in the ends of the hair, making it difficult
    to check the line?
    a. Cutting comb.   c. Wide-tooth comb.
    b. Classic styling brush.   d. Round brush.   ____

17. Once the blunt cut is dry, what type of line should you see?
   a. Even, horizontal line all the way around the head.
   b. Central vertical line from crown to occipital.
   c. Line parallel to the parting.
   d. Slight arc-shaped line.   ____

18. For the graduated cut, in preparation for _____, you should create a radial section by taking a radial parting from the crown to the top of each ear.
   a. razor cutting   c. texturizing
   b. layering   d. tapering   ____

19. What should you do for a graduated cut once the hair is dry?
   a. Detangle the hair with the wide-tooth comb.
   b. Texturize the interior.
   c. Detail the perimeter.
   d. Comb the hair to natural fall.   ____

20. For the uniform-layered cut, how should you dry the hair?
   a. Naturally.   c. Blowdryer.
   b. With your hands.   d. Diffuser.   ____

21. For the uniform-layered haircut, once dry, you should texturize the interior to remove weight by using _____.
   a. razor cutting   c. carving
   b. slithering   d. deep point cutting ____

22. Clients with long hair want to see their length at the _____.
   a. front and back   c. sideburn area
   b. just in front of the ear d. the sides   ____

23. For a long-layered cut, section the hair the same way it was cut and blowdry using a _____.
   a. classic styling brush   c. wide-toothed comb
   b. large round brush   d. styling comb   ____

24. For a long-layered cut, _____ the haircut by taking a horizontal section at the top and looking for an increase in length.
   a. detail   c. cross-check
   b. graduate   d. style   ____

25. For a long-layered cut, the thickness of the hair section you work with may vary due to hair _____.
   a. density   c. porosity
   b. texture   d. length   ____

17 CHEMICAL TEXTURE SERVICES

MULTIPLE CHOICE

1. The chemical hair relaxing process includes a(n)
   _____.
   a. lightener
   b. neutralizer
   c. end paper
   d. perm rod ____

2. Which of the following is also known as a Jheri® curl?
   a. Water waving.
   b. Permanent waving.
   c. Curl reformation.
   d. Chemical hair relaxing. ____

3. Permanent waving _____.
   a. rearranges the basic structure of overly curly hair into
      a straighter hair form
   b. restructures very curly hair into a larger curl pattern
   c. decreases the fullness of fine, softer hair
   d. redirects resistant growth patterns until new
      growth occurs ____

4. Pictures, magazines, and stylebooks help you to figure out
   the client's _____.
   a. likes and dislikes
   b. spending habits
   c. lifestyle
   d. level of confidence ____

5. What type of questions will help you to determine the client's
   desires and past experience with texture services?
   a. Open-ended.
   b. Closed.
   c. Rhetorical.
   d. Casual. ____

6. How long will a client consultation typically take?
   a. A few minutes.
   b. A half hour.
   c. An hour.
   d. A full appointment. ____

7. What type of hair has a raised cuticle layer that easily
   absorbs chemical solutions?
   a. Dense.
   b. Coarse.
   c. Resistant.
   d. Porous. ____

8. If the elasticity is good, the hair _____ after stretching.
   a. expands
   b. contracts
   c. tangles
   d. curls
   ____

9. What type of hair may be more resistant to chemical processes?
   a. Porous.
   b. Medium.
   c. Coarse.
   d. Fine.
   ____

10. Hair _____ describes the diameter of a single strand of hair as being coarse, medium, or fine.
   a. texture
   b. density
   c. porosity
   d. elasticity
   ____

11. Do not proceed with the chemical service if the hair shows signs of _____ .
   a. stretching
   b. whorls
   c. porosity
   d. breakage
   ____

12. Which of the following layers of hair gives the hair its strength, flexibility, elasticity, and shape?
   a. Medulla.
   b. Cortex.
   c. Protein.
   d. Cuticle.
   ____

13. Thio relaxing products require the use of a(n) _____ to chemically oxidize the hair.
   a. moisturizer
   b. activator
   c. neutralizer
   d. texturizer
   ____

14. Hydroxide relaxers can have a pH as high as _____ .
   a. 9.0
   b. 9.6
   c. 10.0
   d. 13.5
   ____

15. Waving lotions/solutions break the disulfide bonds, which is called _____ .
   a. reformation
   b. oxidation
   c. reduction
   d. lanthionization
   ____

16. What type of substances used in chemical texture products break chemical bonds and allow for softening and expansion of the hair?
   a. Mercaptamine.
   b. Alkaline.
   c. Acidic.
   d. Alkanolamine.
   ____

17. _____are strong alkalis that can swell the hair up to twice its normal diameter.

    a. Thio relaxers

    b. Waving solutions

    c. Neutralizers

    d. Hydroxide relaxers   ____

18. Amino acids form proteins, and chemical reactions among proteins produce _____.

    a. peptide linkages

    b. ammonium sulfites

    c. glyceryl monothioglycolates

    d. alkaline substances   ____

19. In the cortex layer, the hair develops and maintains its natural form by means of the physical and chemical _____.

    a. penetration

    b. reactions

    c. concentrations

    d. cross-bonds   ____

20. Cysteine is a(n)_____ obtained by the reduction of cystine.

    a. alkali

    b. amino acid

    c. oxidizing agent

    d. reducing agent   ____

21. Which of the following is the most commonly used perm rod?

    a. Loop.

    b. Straight.

    c. Concave.

    d. Bender.   ____

22. The _____ wrap uses one paper folded in half over the ends of the hair.

    a. bookend

    b. double-end

    c. single flat

    d. double flat   ____

23. What type of rod is used when a definite wave pattern, close to the head, is desired?

    a. Straight.

    b. Circle tool.

    c. Bender.

    d. Concave.   ____

24. The _____ rod is a plastic-coated tool measuring about 12 inches with a uniform diameter along the length of the rod.

    a. concave

    b. circle

    c. bender

    d. concave   ____

25. Which of the following is used to secure the hair and the rod into the desired position to prevent the curl from unwinding during a procedure?

    a. Elastic band.

    b. Stiff wires.

    c. Fastening the ends.

    d. Absorbent papers.   ____

26. What wrap can be used with short rods or short lengths of hair?

    a. Double-flat.
    c. Bookend.

    b. Single-end.
    d. Double-end.   ____

27. _____ are effective in helping to smooth out the wrapping of uneven hair lengths.

    a. Conditioners
    c. Fishhooks

    b. Relaxers
    d. End papers   ____

28. What type of rod is usually used for a body wave that serves as a foundation for further styling?

    a. Bender.
    c. Circle tool.

    b. Large and straight.
    d. Concave.   ____

29. What type of rod creates a consistently sized wave from one side of the hair parting to the other?

    a. Concave.
    c. Bender.

    b. Straight.
    d. Loop.   ____

30. With what wrapping method may it be difficult to control the hair?

    a. Single-end.
    c. Double flat.

    b. Bookend.
    d. Double-end.   ____

31. _____ refers to the position of the perm rod or tool in relation to its base section.

    a. Wrapping pattern
    c. Base control

    b. Wave formation
    d. Base direction   ____

32. Half off-base placement results in _____.

    a. maximum movement

    b. medium volume and movement

    c. greater volume at the scalp area

    d. the least amount of volume and movement   ____

33. On-base placement refers to when the hair is projected about _____ beyond perpendicular.

    a. 30 degrees
    c. 90 degrees

    b. 45 degrees
    d. 180 degrees   ____

34. When using the _____ perm wrap technique, the hair is wound from the hair ends toward the scalp.

    a. croquignole
    c. water

    b. spiral
    d. lotion   ____

35. What type of rod is usually used for a spiral wrap?
- **a.** Bender.
- **b.** Concave.
- **c.** Straight.
- **d.** Loop.

_____

36. What type of perm wrap is appropriate for long hair designs and produces a uniform curl formation from the scalp to the ends?
- **a.** Croquignole.
- **b.** Bookend.
- **c.** Water.
- **d.** Spiral.

_____

37. What type of wrapping pattern is best to use for men's styles, as it produces a more natural-looking wave pattern?
- **a.** Basic.
- **b.** Curvature.
- **c.** Bricklay.
- **d** Piggyback.

_____

38. The _____ perm pattern will blend hair from one area to another.
- **a.** bricklay
- **b.** curvature
- **c.** piggyback
- **d.** basic

_____

39. In what wrapping pattern are all the rods within a panel positioned in the same direction on equal-size bases?
- **a.** Piggyback.
- **b.** Bricklay.
- **c.** Basic.
- **d.** Curvature.

_____

40. Zigzag partings are also known as the _____ technique.
- **a.** textured
- **b.** spiral
- **c.** bricklay
- **d.** weave

_____

41. Perm wraps begin with sectioning the hair into _____.
- **a.** patterns
- **b.** bands
- **c.** panels
- **d.** contours

_____

42. What type of perm wrap uses two perm rods for each parting of hair to create even curl formation on long and/or dense hair?
- **a.** Bricklay.
- **b.** Curvature.
- **c.** Basic.
- **d.** Piggyback.

_____

43. For fine hair, the diameter of the rod will be _____.
- **a.** thick
- **b.** small
- **c.** large
- **d.** medium

_____

44. What type of technique increases the size of the curl as it nears the scalp area, with a tighter curl at the ends?
   a. Croquignole perm wrap.
   b. Spiral wrapping.
   c. Bookend wrapping.
   d. Double-end wrapping. ____

45. The main active ingredient or reducing agent in alkaline perms is _____ .
   a. alkanolamines
   b. hydrogen peroxide
   c. ammonium thioglycolate
   d. glyceryl monothioglycolate ____

46. What type of waves requires the use of an outside heat source to activate chemical reactions and processing?
   a. Cold.   c. Exothermic.
   b. Acid-balanced.   d. Endothermic. ____

47. Which of the following results in a limp or weak wave formation with undefined ridges within the S pattern?
   a. Faster processing.
   b. Underprocessing.
   c. Reconditioning.
   d. Overprocessing. ____

48. One of the benefits associated with alkaline perms are _____ .
   a. strong curl patterns
   b. softer curl patterns
   c. slower, but more controllable processing times
   d. gentler treatment for delicate hair types ____

49. Ammonia-free waves use _____ to replace ammonia.
   a. alkanolamines   c. cysteamines
   b. mercaptamines   d. bisulfites ____

50. A resistant strength of permanent waving products can be used on what type of hair?
   a. Tinted hair.   c. Damaged hair.
   b. Hair with less porosity. d. Porous hair. ____

51. What type of hydroxide relaxer is known as a lye relaxer?
   a. Calcium.   c. Sodium.
   b. Guanidine. d. Lithium. ____

52. Calcium hydroxide relaxers require the addition of a(n)_____.

    a. moisturizer   **c.** conditioner

    b. neutralizer   **d.** activator   ____

53. Which of the following is the oldest and most commonly used chemical relaxer?

    a. Guanidine hydroxide.   **c.** Thio.

    b. Sodium hydroxide.   **d.** Lithium hydroxide.   ____

54. No-base relaxers contain a base cream that is designed to _____ at body temperature.

    a. melt   **c.** be absorbed

    b. harden   **d.** evaporate   ____

55. What type of relaxer is sold in *base* and *no-base* formulas?

    a. Thio.

    b. Chemical neutralizing.

    c. Ammonium thioglycolate.

    d. Hydroxide.   ____

56. What type of strand test is used for determining the hair's reaction to the chemical and processing time?

    a. Elasticity.   **c.** Porosity.

    b. Relaxer.   **d.** Density.   ____

57. For a relaxer strand test, thread a small section of hair through a hole cut into a piece of wax paper or paper towel, and do not use _____.

    a. neutralizing shampoo   **c.** foil

    b. neutralizer   **d.** water   ____

58. The thio relaxer product used for the partial relaxation of the hair in a curl reformation service is known as the _____.

    a. weave   **c.** booster

    b. neutralizer   **d.** rearranger   ____

59. In curl reformation, what solution rebuilds the broken disulfide bonds?

    a. Neutralizer.   **c.** Rearranger.

    b. Booster.   **d.** Waving.   ____

60. In curl reformation, what chemical restructures the hair around perm rods?

    a. Neutralizer.   **c.** Booster.

    b. Rearranger.   **d.** Activator.   ____

61. What type of styling product is often recommended as part of the finishing process of a curl reformation?
   a. Pomade.
   c. Texturizer.
   b. Moisturizer.
   d. Conditioner. _____

62. The rearranger is an ATG product in a _____ form.
   a. foam
   c. spray liquid
   b. powder
   d. thick cream _____

63. Relaxing products can be used to _____.
   a. protect and control the ends of the hair
   b. texturize the hair
   c. wrap the hair
   d. create volume and lift _____

64. Sodium hydroxide is an extremely _____ product.
   a. alkaline
   c. porous
   b. acidic
   d. overprocessed _____

65. What type of service is used to eliminate up to 95 percent of frizz and curl, lasts three to five months, and may cause health risks if not performed properly?
   a. Calcium hydroxide relaxer.
   b. Thio relaxer.
   c. Keratin-based treatment.
   d. No-base relaxer. _____

66. A _____ service partially straightens the hair with the intent that it will be picked out and cut.
   a. curl reformation
   b. retouch
   c. keratin-based straightening
   d. chemical blowout _____

67. Thio relaxers may have a pH of _____.
   a. between 4.5 and 7.0
   b. between 7.8 and 8.2
   c. between 9.0 and 9.6
   d. above 10 _____

68. The objective of a chemical blowout is to remove some but not all of the _____.
   a. body
   c. moisture
   b. curl
   d. elasticity _____

69. Texturizers and chemical blowouts are usually performed with a _____ relaxer.
   a. potassium hydroxide
   c. lithium hydroxide
   b. guanidine hydroxide
   d. thio
   ____

70. After a chemical blowout, the final cutting will be done with _____ to even out loose or ragged ends.
   a. a trimmer
   c. shears
   b. a razor
   d. clippers
   ____

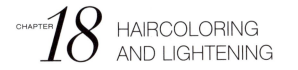

CHAPTER 18 HAIRCOLORING AND LIGHTENING

MULTIPLE CHOICE

1. What type of hair has melanin granules grouped tightly?
   - **a.** Fine.
   - **b.** Coarse.
   - **c.** Medium-textured.
   - **d.** Curly. ____

2. What determines the hair's ability to absorb haircolor products?
   - **a.** Density.
   - **b.** Texture.
   - **c.** Porosity.
   - **d.** Elasticity. ____

3. What color hair is the result of a reduction in the production of melanin pigments?
   - **a.** Light blond.
   - **b.** White.
   - **c.** Dark blond.
   - **d.** Gray. ____

4. Which of the following provides natural black and brown pigment (color) to hair?
   - **a.** Derivatives.
   - **b.** Eumelanin.
   - **c.** Keratin.
   - **d.** Pheomelanin. ____

5. _____ is an indication of the strength of the hair's cortex.
   - **a.** Porosity
   - **b.** Elasticity
   - **c.** Density
   - **d.** Texture ____

6. If the cuticle is tight, making the hair more resistant to chemical penetration, this indicates what type of porosity?
   - **a.** High.
   - **b.** Medium.
   - **c.** Low.
   - **d.** Average. ____

7. White hair is actually the color of keratin without _____.
   - **a.** eumelanin
   - **b.** base color
   - **c.** pheomelanin
   - **d.** melanin ____

8. What is indicated by wet hair that does not return to its original length when stretched?
   - **a.** Low elasticity.
   - **b.** High porosity.
   - **c.** Normal elasticity.
   - **d.** Low porosity. ____

9. During a porosity test, if you feel a slight roughness to the hair, it is considered _____ porosity.
   a. low
   b. dense
   c. average
   d. high ____

10. What type of pigment is the pigment that lies under the natural hair color?
   a. Natural.
   b. Contributing.
   c. Foundational.
   d. Artificial. ____

11. The three primary colors are yellow, red, and _____.
   a. gray
   b. white
   c. blue
   d. black ____

12. Which of the following is the weakest of the primary colors and will lighten and brighten other colors?
   a. Red.
   b. White.
   c. Blue.
   d. Yellow. ____

13. What type of colors are created by mixing equal amounts of two primary colors?
   a. Secondary.
   b. Tertiary.
   c. Complementary.
   d. Quaternary. ____

14. An example of a tertiary color would be _____.
   a. violet
   b. yellow-green
   c. orange
   d. yellow and violet ____

15. When mixed together, complementary colors _____ each other.
   a. brighten
   b. neutralize
   c. highlight
   d. intensify ____

16. The _____ color of a haircoloring product is the predominant tone of a color.
   a. complementary
   b. natural
   c. base
   d. primary ____

17. Which of the following describes the warmth or coolness of a color?
   a. Natural level.
   b. Intensity.
   c. Hue.
   d. Tone. ____

18. A neutral base color tends to _____ .
   a. soften and balance other colors
   b. produce cool results
   c. create warm, bright tones in the hair
   d. minimize yellow tones   ____

19. Which of the following would be considered a warm color?
   a. Violet.   **c.** Blue.
   b. Green.   **d.** Red.   ____

20. What type of nonoxidizing haircolor washes out or fades within a few weeks?
   a. Demipermanent.   **c.** Temporary.
   b. Permanent.   **d.** Semipermanent.   ____

21. A demipermanent color would do which of the following?
   a. Add subtle color results.
   b. Act as a filler in color correction.
   c. Neutralize yellow or other unwanted tones.
   d. Create fun, bold results that easily shampoo from the hair.   ____

22. If you wanted to introduce a client to haircolor services, you would use what type of haircolor?
   a. Demipermanent.   **c.** Semipermanent.
   b. Temporary.   **d.** Permanent.   ____

23. What serves as the main oxidizing agent used in haircoloring?
   a. Hydrogen peroxide.   **c.** Bleach.
   b. Aniline derivatives.   **d.** Metallic salts.   ____

24. Compound dyes are metallic or mineral dyes combined with a _____ .
   a. solvent   **c.** vegetable tint
   b. synthetic wax   **d.** diffused melanin   ____

25. Which of the following is not a professional haircoloring product?
   a. Amino tint.   **c.** Vegetable tint.
   b. Metallic dye.   **d.** Synthetic-organic tint.   ____

26. An example of a vegetable tint would be _____ .
   a. a color restorer   **c.** aniline derivative tints
   b. a progressive color   **d.** henna   ____

27. Which of the following would be another term for an activator?
    a. Accelerator.
    b. Lightener.
    c. Developer.
    d. Generator.
    ____

28. 20-volume hydrogen peroxide would be used _____.
    a. with demipermanent products to deposit color
    b. when less lightening is desired
    c. with permanent color products to cover gray
    d. with permanent haircolor to achieve up to three levels of lift/lightening in one step
    ____

29. Permanent haircolor products are alkaline and range between _____ on the pH scale.
    a. 2.0 and 4.5
    b. 3.5 and 4.0
    c. 7.0 and 9.0
    d. 9.0 and 10.5
    ____

30. As soon as hydrogen peroxide is mixed into the lightener formula, it begins to release _____.
    a. an alkaline agent
    b. nitrogen
    c. oxygen
    d. hydrogen
    ____

31. _____ lighteners add temporary color as they lighten.
    a. Neutral oil
    b. Powder
    c. Cream
    d. Color oil
    ____

32. _____ hair will absorb the base color of the toner.
    a. Overlightened
    b. Pre-lightened
    c. Gray
    d. Underlightened
    ____

33. Which of the following is designed to correct excessive porosity?
    a. Solvents.
    b. Fillers.
    c. Removers.
    d. Toners.
    ____

34. Toners are only applied to what type of hair?
    a. Underlightened.
    b. Blond.
    c. Pre-lightened.
    d. Overlightened.
    ____

35. Cream lighteners contain conditioning agents called _____ agents.
    a. bluing
    b. swelling
    c. oxidizing
    d. alkaline
    ____

36. Color fillers use certified colors as _____.
    a. treatments   **c.** hues
    b. pigments   **d.** activators   ____

37. Which of the following would be an example of single-process coloring?
    a. The hair is lightened.
    b. Cap frost.
    c. A depositing color is applied.
    d. Tint retouch applications.   ____

38. _____ is the process of coloring strands or sections of the hair darker than the natural or artificial color.
    a. Highlighting   **c.** Lowlighting
    b. Pre-softening   **d.** Retouching   ____

39. What type of lighting is not suitable for judging existing hair colors?
    a. Incandescent.   **c.** Strong natural light.
    b. Well-lit room.   **d.** Fluorescent.   ____

40. A(n) _____ application is the application of haircolor to hair that has not been previously colored.
    a. toner   **c.** virgin
    b. single   **d.** on-the-scalp   ____

41. What type of test is given 24 to 48 hours prior to each application of an aniline derivative tint or toner?
    a. Metallic salt.   **c.** Porosity.
    b. Strand.   **d.** Patch.   ____

42. _____ is the process of coloring hair back to its natural color.
    a. Single-process haircoloring   **c.** Retouching
    b. Tint back   **d.** Pre-softening   ____

43. In which of the following techniques do you paint a lightener or color directly onto clean, styled hair?
    a. Free-form.   **c.** Cap frost.
    b. Foil frost.   **d.** Streaking.   ____

44. Soap caps can be used to _____.
    a. facilitate better color penetration
    b. color hair back to its natural color
    c. reduce unwanted yellow tones in gray hair
    d. add the illusion of sheen and depth to hair   ____

45. Temporary color rinses can be used to _____.
   a. remove undesirable casts and off-shades
   b. darken the hair and cover gray
   c. paint, streak, or frost certain sections of the hair
   d. tone down overlightened hair   ____

46. With what type of color will hair usually return to its natural
   color after six to eight shampoos?
   a. Semipermanent.   c. Demipermanent.
   b. Temporary.   d. Permanent.   ____

47. What is one of the most important characteristics to
   consider when choosing hair color tint shades?
   a. Texture.   c. Density.
   b. Porosity.   d. Elasticity.   ____

48. Double-process haircoloring begins with hair _____.
   a. tinting   c. lightening
   b. toner   d. shampooing   ____

49. Hair lighteners can be used to _____.
   a. temporarily restore faded hair color to its natural shade
   b. neutralize yellow tones in white or gray hair
   c. tone down overlightened hair
   d. remove undesirable casts and off-shades   ____

50. Which of the following are formulated specifically for
   coloring mustaches and beards?
   a. Pomades.   c. Metallic dyes.
   b. Aniline derivative tints.   d. Progressive dyes.   ____

51. What should never be used for coloring mustaches?
   a. Liquid tints.   c. Aniline derivative tints.
   b. Hair color crayons.   d. Pomades.   ____

52. To restore damaged hair to a healthier condition, hair
   conditioners containing _____ substances should be
   used.
   a. eumelanin   c. pheomelanin
   b. lanolin   d. an aniline derivative   ____

53. Gray, white, and salt-and-pepper hair with a yellowish cast
   can be treated with _____ colors.
   a. blue-based   c. red-based
   b. green-based   d. violet-based   ____

54. Which of the following have been known to cause severe allergic reactions when applied to facial hair or around freshly cut hairlines?
a. Hair color crayons.
b. Liquid eyebrow and eyelash tints.
c. Pomades.
d. Metallic or progressive dyes. ____

55. Because there is no _____ in the hair, gray hair may appear lighter after haircolor is applied.
a. protein
b. melanin
c. keratin
d. lanolin ____

56. Some gray hair tends to be resistant to chemical processes and may require _____ before a service.
a. pre-lightening
b. shampooing
c. pre-softening
d. a predisposition test ____

57. What type of tones indicates overlightening?
a. Ash.
b. Gold.
c. Red.
d. Violet. ____

58. Gray hair and skin tone changes that accompany advancing years may benefit from _____ tones.
a. gold
b. red
c. silver
d. beige ____

59. What type of lighteners are the mildest form of lightener?
a. Powder.
b. Cream.
c. Virgin.
d. Oil. ____

60. When working with a cream or paste lightener, it must be the thickness of _____ .
a. heavy wax
b. whipped cream
c. shampoo
d. gel ____

61. Cap all bottles of developer and lightener to avoid _____ .
a. loss of strength
b. breathing in vapors
c. dripping
d. skin irritation ____

62. Do not apply tint if a patch test is _____ .
a. negative
b. complete
c. positive
d. neutral ____

63. Choose a shade of tint that harmonizes with the client's _____ .

    a. favorite color   **c.** eyes

    b. personality   **d.** complexion   ____

64. What temperature should the water be for removing tint?

    a. Lukewarm.   **c.** Cold.

    b. Very hot.   **d.** ice cold.   ____

65. What should you not do prior to a tint?

    a. Examine the scalp.   **c.** Perform a strand test.

    b. Perform a patch test.   **d.** Brush the hair.   ____

19 PREPARING FOR LICENSURE AND EMPLOYMENT

MULTIPLE CHOICE

1. Being _____ means understanding the strategies for successfully taking tests.
   - **a.** trained
   - **b.** test-wise
   - **c.** skilled
   - **d.** able to memorize
      ____

2. The most important factor that will affect your test performance is your _____.
   - **a.** physical state
   - **b.** time management skill
   - **c.** mastery of course content
   - **d.** psychological state
      ____

3. What should you avoid the night before an examination?
   - **a.** Test-taking strategies.
   - **b.** Reviewing handouts.
   - **c.** Rest.
   - **d.** Cramming.
      ____

4. On the exam, what questions should you answer first?
   - **a.** The easiest ones.
   - **b.** The most difficult ones.
   - **c.** The shortest ones.
   - **d.** The longest ones.
      ____

5. Which of the following is the basic question or problem?
   - **a.** Key word.
   - **b.** Choice.
   - **c.** Stem.
   - **d.** Statement.
      ____

6. In multiple choice questions, when two choices are close or similar, _____.
   - **a.** both could be right
   - **b.** both should be eliminated
   - **c.** one of them is probably wrong
   - **d.** one of them is probably right
      ____

7. In multiple choice questions, if there is no penalty, what should do if you do not know the answer?
   - **a.** Guess.
   - **b.** Do not answer the question.
   - **c.** Answer all as correct.
   - **d.** Mark the two choices that may be correct.
      ____

8. For true/false questions, what should you look for?
   a. Absolute words.
   c. Related words.
   b. Qualifying words.
   d. Similar words. ____

9. What type of reasoning is the process of reaching logical conclusions by employing logical reasoning?
   a. Relative.
   c. Deductive.
   b. Effective.
   d. Objective. ____

10. Basic preparation for practical exams should always include _____ .
   a. well-organized notes
   b. new technologies
   c. professional references
   d. practice on the model you are taking ____

11. For what type of question should you organize your answer according to the cue words in the question?
   a. Multiple choice.
   c. Essay.
   b. True/False.
   d. Matching. ____

12. In addition to testing basic theory concepts, the written exam contains questions about your _____ .
   a. performance
   b. primary goals
   c. strongest practical skills
   d. state's barber laws and rules ____

13. When you have _____ , you are committed to a strong code of moral and artistic values.
   a. good technical skills
   b. integrity
   c. a strong work ethic
   d. motivation ____

14. The best kind of motivation is _____ .
   a. internal
   c. team-related
   b. peer pressure
   d. parental pressure ____

15. The average time a potential employer will spend scanning your resume before deciding to grant you an interview is about _____ .
   a. 20 seconds
   c. 1 minute
   b. 45 seconds
   d. 5 minutes ____

16. What should you stress on your resume?
    a. Information on why you left prior employer.
    b. Personal information.
    c. Salary requirements.
    d. Accomplishments. ____

17. What type of skill is mastered at other jobs, and then can be put to use in a new position?
    a. Transferable.   **c.** Test-taking.
    b. Career.   **d.** Academic. ____

18. A great way to find out about potential jobs is to _____.
    a. wait until you graduate
    b. network
    c. complete an inventory of personal characteristics
    d. hire someone to assist you ____

19. On your resume, what type of statement enlarges your basic duties and responsibilities?
    a. Relevant.   **c.** Qualifying.
    b. Positive.   **d.** Accomplishment. ____

20. In the barbering business, having a(n) _____ means taking pride in your work and committing yourself to consistently doing a good job.
    a. strong code of moral values
    b. enthusiastic nature
    c. strong work ethic
    d. attractive appearance ____

21. Which of the following is possibly the least expensive way of owning your own business?
    a. Regional franchise shop.
    b. Spa.
    c. Independent local chain.
    d. Booth rental. ____

22. A _____ is a written summary of a person's education and work experience.
    a. cover letter   **c.** portfolio
    b. resume   **d.** template ____

23. Do not state _____ on your resume.
    a. your salary history
    b. professional references
    c. past accomplishments
    d. skills mastered at other jobs ____

24. On your resume, you should begin accomplishment statements with _____.
    a. key words
    b. absolutes
    c. action verbs
    d. qualifying words ____

25. Which of the following is the compass that keeps you on course over the long haul of your career?
    a. Ability.
    b. Integrity.
    c. Opportunity.
    d. Versatility. ____

26. What should you always include with your resume?
    a. Cover letter.
    b. Salary references.
    c. Information about why you left former positions.
    d. Flowery language. ____

27. Remember to follow up the interview with a _____.
    a. request for a second interview
    b. request for a job offer
    c. thank-you note
    d. thank-you gift ____

28. During the interview, questions regarding _____ are permitted.
    a. date-of-birth
    b. disabilities
    c. medical conditions
    d. drug or tobacco use ____

29. During the interview, it is legal to ask if the applicant is _____.
    a. younger than 18
    b. disabled
    c. a native Spanish speaker
    d. a U.S. citizen ____

30. Any time you are applying for a position, you will be required to complete a(n) _____.
    a. resume
    b. application
    c. portfolio
    d. cover letter ____

31. What type of agreement prohibits you from seeking employment within a given time period and geographic area after you leave employment with your current employer?
    a. Apprenticeship.
    b. Noncompete.
    c. Confidentiality.
    d. Training. ____

32. Which of the following would be a typical question asked during a proper interview?
    a. Are you a U.S. citizen?
    b. How old are you?
    c. What skills do you feel are your strongest?
    d. What is your native language? ____

33. Which of these questions is a legal question to ask during an interview?
    a. What is your marital status?
    b. Do you have any children?
    c. Are you a U.S. citizen?
    d. Are you physically able to perform this job? ____

34. An employer may obtain the applicant's agreement to _____ .
    a. submit to drug testing
    b. be a citizen of the U.S.
    c. disclose his or her sexual orientation
    d. request his or her medical records ____

35. During an interview, answer questions honestly and do not speak for more than _____ at a time.
    a. 30 seconds
    b. 1 minute
    c. 2 minutes
    d. 5 minutes ____

36. _____ is the universal language.
    a. A good first impression
    b. English
    c. Hand shaking
    d. Smiling ____

37. Some barbershops require applicants to _____ as part of the interview.
    a. role play
    b. perform a service in their chosen discipline
    c. complete medical history forms
    d. answer illegal questions ____

38. The _____ prohibits general inquiries about health problems, disabilities, and medical conditions.
    a. Americans with Disabilities Act
    b. State Board Exam
    c. Labor Law
    d. Social Security Administration ____

39. During an interview, you should close with a(n) _____ statement that you want the job (if you do).
   a. positive
   b. accomplishment
   c. qualifying
   d. relevant   ____

40. Who benefits from a noncompete agreement?
   a. Student.
   b. Client.
   c. Business owner.
   d. Employee.   ____

20 WORKING BEHIND THE CHAIR

MULTIPLE CHOICE

1. Barbering school is a _____ environment.
   - **a.** commission-paying
   - **b.** team
   - **c.** forgiving
   - **d.** marketing ____

2. Working in a barbershop requires each staff member to work as a(n) _____ .
   - **a.** booth renter
   - **b.** team member
   - **c.** mentor
   - **d.** educator ____

3. Which of the following is central to the barbering business?
   - **a.** Scheduling.
   - **b.** High-paying commissions.
   - **c.** Getting ahead.
   - **d.** Web resources. ____

4. You should be true to your word by choosing your words carefully and _____ .
   - **a.** automatically
   - **b.** precisely
   - **c.** efficiently
   - **d.** honestly ____

5. Which of the following is the key to teamwork?
   - **a.** Communication.
   - **b.** Competition.
   - **c.** Ambition.
   - **d.** Determination. ____

6. Working as an independent contractor and working as a booth renter are forms of _____ .
   - **a.** being a role model
   - **b.** being an employee
   - **c.** self-employment
   - **d.** self-confidence ____

7. In a(n) _____ compensation structure, the employer pays you a percentage of the gross service sales you generate.
   - **a.** straight salary
   - **b.** hourly salary
   - **c.** salary-plus-commission
   - **d.** commission ____

8. A salary-plus-commission compensation arrangement is sometimes called a(n) _____.
   a. upsell
   b. guarantee
   c. default
   d. percentage ____

9. In a _____ arrangement, you are actually setting up a small business.
   a. fixed salary
   b. guarantee
   c. booth rental
   d. commission-only ____

10. Commission is usually offered once an employee has _____.
    a. trusted coworkers
    b. a personal financial budget in place
    c. completed barbering school
    d. built a loyal clientele ____

11. Tips are income and must be tracked and reported on your _____.
    a. monthly budget worksheet
    b. income tax return
    c. individual retirement account
    d. daily log ____

12. Not paying back your loans is called _____.
    a. defaulting
    b. charging
    c. borrowing
    d. forgiving ____

13. The best way to record your tips and additional income is to _____.
    a. have an accountant
    b. have a financial planner
    c. keep a daily log
    d. keep a budget worksheet ____

14. Which of the following is the act of recommending and selling products to your clients for at-home use?
    a. Servicing.
    b. Ticket upgrading.
    c. Upselling.
    d. Retailing. ____

15. You should be _____ when recommending products for sale.
    a. self-confident
    b. self-employed
    c. emphatic
    d. hard selling ____

16. Keep in mind that the best interests of _____ should be your first consideration.
    a. the barbershop
    b. the client
    c. yourself
    d. suppliers   ____

17. Which of the following is now the preferred mode of communication for many people?
    a. Social media.
    b. Mail.
    c. Telephone.
    d. E-mail.   ____

18. Being _____ means that you do not gossip or make fun of anyone or anything related to the barbershop.
    a. successful
    b. resentful
    c. respectful
    d. honest   ____

19. Providing _____ must always be your first concern.
    a. good financial compensation
    b. additional products
    c. good-quality service
    d. a good understanding of what is expected of you   ____

20. What form of advertisement is not expensive, and is always greatly appreciated?
    a. Public speaking.
    b. Local business referrals.
    c. Business card referrals.
    d. Birthday cards.   ____

21 THE BUSINESS OF BARBERING

MULTIPLE CHOICE

1. Barbershop owners have no guarantee of _____ .
   a. credit
   b. profits
   c. services
   d. support
   ____

2. Owning your own barbershop or renting a booth in an existing shop or salon requires _____ .
   a. familiarity with building codes
   b. a business partnership
   c. a strong line of credit
   d. community outreach
   ____

3. Which of the following is a guide to the actions of the organization?
   a. Mission statement.
   b. Goals.
   c. Vision statement.
   d. Business plan.
   ____

4. What business time period would be appropriate for adding more locations or expanding the scope of the business?
   a. Years 1 to 3.
   b. Years 2 to 5.
   c. Years 5 to 10.
   d. Years 11 to 20.
   ____

5. A _____ is a written description of your business as you see it today and as you foresee it in the next 5 years.
   a. benchmark
   b. written agreement
   c. business plan
   d. brand identity
   ____

6. Which of the following is an ownership structure controlled by one or more stockholders?
   a. Franchise.
   b. Corporation.
   c. Partnership.
   d. Sole proprietor.
   ____

7. One reason for going into a partnership arrangement is to
   _____ .
   a. have the last say in decision making
   b. have a known name and brand recognition
   c. have help running your operation
   d. maintain a corporate status ____

8. One of the requirements for a partnership arrangement is
   _____ .
   a. having stockholders
   b. paying unemployment insurance taxes
   c. promoting, protecting, and furthering the interests of
      businesses in a community
   d. trust ____

9. In a business plan, the owner's resume and personal
   financial information would be found in the _____ .
   a. supporting documents
   b. financial documents
   c. vision statement
   d. executive summary ____

10. The kinds of services your business will offer and the quality
    of those services is found in what part of the business plan?
    a. Marketing plan.
    b. Vision statement.
    c. Mission statement.
    d. Organizational plan. ____

11. Supplies that are used in the daily business operation are
    _____ supplies.
    a. service   c. merchandise
    b. consumption   d. retail ____

12. Someone who is trained to do everything from recording
    sales and payroll to generating a profit-and-loss statement is
    called a(n) _____ .
    a. stockholder   c. receptionist
    b. business manager   d. full-charge bookkeeper ____

13. Unless you are at least _____ booked all the time, it
    may not be advantageous to rent a booth.
    a. 50 percent   c. 70 percent
    b. 60 percent   d. 95 percent ____

14. In how many states is booth rental not allowed?
    a. 0.
    b. 2.
    c. 20.
    d. 50.
    ____

15. What should be the primary concern when constructing the best physical layout for a barbershop?
    a. Cost.
    b. Personnel.
    c. Retail sales.
    d. Maximum efficiency.
    ____

16. How long does it take for most new shops to begin operating at full capacity?
    a. 3 months.
    b. 6 months.
    c. 1 year.
    d. 2 years.
    ____

17. Which of the following is considered a barbershop's nerve center?
    a. Reception area.
    b. Booth spaces.
    c. Break room.
    d. Shampoo area.
    ____

18. An advertising budget should not exceed _____ of your gross income.
    a. 3 percent
    b. 5 percent
    c. 10 percent
    d. 12 percent
    ____

19. The first goal of every business should be to _____.
    a. add more services
    b. sell retail products
    c. upsell your clients
    d. maintain current clients
    ____

20. Which of the following is the best form of advertising?
    a. Social media.
    b. Satisfied clients.
    c. Television advertising.
    d. Giveaway promotional items.
    ____

SAMPLE STATE BOARD
EXAMINATION TEST 1

1. Approaching work with a strong sense of responsibility is an important:
   a. life skill.
   b. self-actualization.
   c. motivation.
   d. personality approach. ____

2. Many primitive cultures had belief systems that elevated tribal barbers to positions of importance, such as:
   a. tonsorial artists.
   b. shamans.
   c. warriors.
   d. rulers. ____

3. A balanced diet includes getting plenty of:
   a. salt.
   b. water.
   c. fats.
   d. sugar. ____

4. The best way to deal with disputes or differences within the barbershop is:
   a. by avoiding the topic.
   b. sharing information with others.
   c. asking questions.
   d. in private. ____

5. Staph bacteria causes:
   a. chicken pox.
   b. influenza.
   c. common colds.
   d. food poisoning. ____

6. An important life skill to remember and practice is:
   a. being helpful and caring to others.
   b. mastering techniques to become more serious.
   c. sticking to goals only if necessary.
   d. maintaining a protective attitude. ____

7. The Latin word _____, meaning "beard," is the origin of the word barber.
   a. *tondere*
   b. *tonsors*
   c. *queue*
   d. *barba* ____

8. Diplococci are spherical bacteria that cause diseases such as:
   a. strep throat.
   b. pneumonia.
   c. syphilis.
   d. typhoid fever. ____

9. Disinfectants are:
   a. pesticides.
   c. germicides.
   b. pathogens.
   d. antiseptics. _____

10. Hepatitis is a bloodborne virus that can damage the:
    a. heart.
    c. lungs.
    b. kidney.
    d. liver. _____

11. To create a mission statement, begin with your:
    a. closest friends.
    b. interests.
    c. educational background.
    d. confidence. _____

12. The Associated Master Barbers and Beauticians of America (AMBBA) adopted the *barber code of ethics* to promote:
    a. professional responsibility.
    b. professional education.
    c. professional licensure.
    d. the profession of beauticians. _____

13. You should never mix bleach with:
    a. detergents.
    c. pesticides.
    b. disinfectants.
    d. water. _____

14. Pathogenic bacteria, viruses, or fungi cannot enter the body through:
    a. the mouth.
    c. the nose.
    b. intact skin.
    d. inflamed skin. _____

15. The acronym NABBA stands for:
    a. National Association of State Board.
    b. National Association of Barber Code.
    c. National Association of Barber Boards of America.
    d. National Association of Barber Code. _____

16. The process used to identify a long-term and short-term goals is:
    a. goal setting.
    c. self-actualization.
    b. mind mapping.
    d. time management. _____

17. In 2010, the barbering fashion trend that returned for young men was:
    a. clean-shaven faces.
    b. sideburns.
    c. long hair.
    d. beards and beard designs. _____

18. All employees should be instructed in how to use:
    a. hydraulic chairs.
    c. implements.
    b. fire extinguishers.
    d. disinfectants. ____

19. Shears that create patterns and texture in hair are:
    a. blending.
    c. thinning.
    b. chunking.
    d. texturing. ____

20. The soap used in electric latherizers is:
    a. liquid cream.
    c. vegetable.
    b. hard.
    d. soft. ____

21 Clear thinking is stimulated by:
    a. note taking.
    b. exercise and recreation.
    c. key words and phrases.
    d. repetition. ____

22. When standing to cut hair, your leg position should be:
    a. at a 30-degree angle.
    c. hip-width apart.
    b. neutral.
    d. bent forwards. ____

23. The invasion of body tissues by disease-causing pathogens is a(n):
    a. infection.
    c. contamination.
    b. disinfection.
    d. fission. ____

24. The weight and length of the blade relative to the handle is razor:
    a. temper.
    c. size.
    b. grind.
    d. balance. ____

25. The study of tiny structures found in living tissues is:
    a. myology.
    c. microscopic anatomy.
    b. physiology.
    d. pathology. ____

26. When taking notes, using key words or phrases helps to identify:
    a. problem-solving activities.
    c. tasks and techniques.
    b. main points.
    d. guidelines. ____

27. As a professional, you should control your emotions and respond rather than:
    a. understand.
    c. disapprove.
    b. react.
    d. listen. ____

28. The tools used for finish and detail work are:
   a. detachable-blade clippers.   **c.** metal combs.
   b. adjustable-blade clippers.   **d.** outliners.   ____

29. Nerve tissue is composed of:
   a. interstitial cells.   **c.** daughter cells.
   b. neurons.   **d.** microscopic cells.   ____

30. The pace preferred when stropping is:
   a. fast.   **c.** uneven.
   b. slow.   **d.** moderate.   ____

31. When you align behavior and actions to values, you are demonstrating:
   a. emotional stability.   **c.** discretion.
   b. integrity.   **d.** diplomacy.   ____

32. Tuberculocidal disinfectants are referred to as:
   a. quats.   **c.** infectious.
   b. nonpathogenic.   **d.** phenolics.   ____

33. You should grasp the towel for a towel wrap:
   a. tautly.   **c.** lengthwise.
   b. vertically.   **d.** loosely.   ____

34. Staphylococci grow in:
   a. strings of beads.
   b. irregular masses.
   c. clusters like bunches of grapes.
   d. pairs.   ____

35. The study of the anatomy, structure, and function of the bones is:
   a. osteology.   **c.** myology.
   b. histology.   **d.** pathology.   ____

36. One benefit of effective communications skills is:
   a. self-promotion.   **c.** self-checks.
   b. self-confidence.   **d.** self-esteem.   ____

37. Pus is a sign of a:
   a. bacterial infection.   **c.** biofilm.
   b. viral infection.   **d.** parasitic infestation.   ____

38. The part of the cell needed for growth, reproduction, and self-repair is the:
   a. cell membrane.
   b. cytoplasm.
   c. protoplasm.
   d. nucleus. _____

39. Sensory nerves are known as:
   a. afferent nerves.
   b. axon nerves.
   c. efferent nerves.
   d. reflex nerves. _____

40. The brain is contained in the:
   a. axon terminal.
   b. cranium.
   c. spinal column.
   d. thorax. _____

41. Laws are written by:
   a. regulatory departments.
   b. federal and state legislatures.
   c. health agencies.
   d. state boards. _____

42. The process that destroys all microbial life including spores is:
   a. cleaning.
   b. sterilization.
   c. sanitizing.
   d. disinfecting. _____

43. The largest bone of the arm that extends from the shoulder to the elbow is the:
   a. humerus.
   b. carpus.
   c. radius.
   d. ulna. _____

44. The word integument means:
   a. bone.
   b. map.
   c. study of.
   d. natural covering. _____

45. Glands that release hormonal secretions directly into the bloodstream are:
   a. duct.
   b. exocrine.
   c. endocrine.
   d. hormonal. _____

46. Chemical products that destroy most bacteria, fungi, and viruses on surfaces are:
   a. disinfectants.
   b. cleansers.
   c. sterilizers.
   d. sanitizers. _____

47. Antiseptics contain a high volume of:
   a. alcohol.
   b. ammonium.
   c. formaldehyde.
   d. sodium hypochlorite. _____

48. Soap in most disinfectants will cause them to become:
a. toxic.
c. inactive.
b. harmful.
d. explosive.
____

49. Clipper guards are known as:
a. attachment combs.
c. edgers.
b. hair shapers.
d. blending shears.
____

50. The machine that introduces water-soluble products into the skin during a facial is:
a. highfrequency.
c. galvanic.
b. tesla.
d. electrotherapy.
____

51. The basic building blocks of all matter are:
a. protons.
c. electrons.
b. molecules.
d. atoms.
____

52. A suspension of one liquid dispersed in another is a(n):
a. emulsion.
c. surfactant.
b. solvent.
d. solution.
____

53. The cationic ingredient used in dandruff shampoos is:
a. sodium laureth sulfate.
b. amphoteric I-20.
c. quaternary ammonium compounds.
d. cocamide.
____

54. The letters pH denote:
a. potential hydrogen.
c. partially hydrophilic.
b. partial hydrogen.
d. potential hydroxide.
____

55. The connection between two or more bones of the skeleton is a:
a. tendon.
c. joint.
b. ligament.
d. nerve.
____

56. The most common element found in the known universe is:
a. hydrogen.
c. sodium.
b. carbon dioxide.
d. oxygen.
____

57. The average pH for hair and skin is:
a. 7.5.
c. 9.0.
b. 3.5.
d. 5.0.
____

58. Astringents have an alcohol content of up to:
a. 4 to 15 percent.
c. 35 percent.
b. 20 percent.
d. 50 percent.
____

59. An example of a good conductor is:
    a. silk.
    b. rubber.
    c. cement.
    d. a watery solution of acid and salt.   ____

60. The color of blood when it is in the veins is:
    a. bright red.   c. light red.
    b. dark red.   d. blue.   ____

61. The loss of oxygen or the addition of hydrogen is:
    a. oxidation.   c. reaction.
    b. reduction.   d. application.   ____

62. You should disconnect an appliance by:
    a. twisting the plug.   c. pulling on the plug.
    b. pulling on the cord.   d. stepping on the cord.   ____

63. The process that introduces water-soluble products into the skin is:
    a. iontophoresis.   c. desincrustation.
    b. anaphoresis.   d. cataphoresis.   ____

64. The light that is known as cold light or actinic light is:
    a. visible.   c. electromagnetic.
    b. infrared.   d. ultraviolet.   ____

65. The nerves that carry impulses from the brain to muscles or glands are:
    a. receptor.   c. motor.
    b. afferent.   d. sensory.   ____

66. Compounds of hydrogen, a metal, and oxygen are:
    a. acids.   c. salts.
    b. oxides.   d. bases.   ____

67. The part of the body where the skin is the thinnest is the:
    a. scalp.   c. hands.
    b. eyelids.   d. shoulders.   ____

68. Sebum secretion is affected by:
    a. heat.   c. pathogens.
    b. injury.   d. hormones.   ____

69. The epidermis contains no:
    a. keratin.   c. melanin.
    b. fibrous protein.   d. blood vessels.   ____

70. The U-shaped bone at the base of the tongue is the:
    a. cervical vertebrae.   c. malar.
    b. mandible.   d. hyoid.   ____

71. Nonaqueous solutions do not have:
    a. volume.   c. shape.
    b. pH.   d. mass.   ____

72. The substance that lubricates the skin and preserves the softness of the hair is:
    a. elastin.   c. melanin.
    b. collagen.   d. sebum.   ____

73. A thick scar resulting from excessive growth of fibrous tissue is a(n):
    a. crust.   c. excoriation.
    b. keloid.   d. cicatrix.   ____

74. The technical term for freckles is:
    a. hypopigmentation.   c. leukoderma.
    b. lentigines.   d. vitiligo.   ____

75. Chemical compounds that attract and retain moisture from the atmosphere are:
    a. fatty alcohols.   c. silicones.
    b. mineral oils.   d. humectants.   ____

76. Moisturizing creams treat:
    a. wrinkles.   c. oil accumulation.
    b. dryness.   d. dandruff.   ____

77. The layer of the dermis that contains the lymph glands is:
    a. reticular.   c. papillary.
    b. basal cell.   d. granular.   ____

78. The vitamin important to skin and tissue repair is:
    a. vitamin A.   c. vitamin C.
    b. vitamin E.   d. vitamin K.   ____

79. A side effect of finasteride is:
    a. a rash.   c. loss of sexual function.
    b. further hair loss.   d. weight loss.   ____

80. The outer layer of the epidermis is the:
    a. stratum lucidum.   c. stratum corneum.
    b. stratum granulosum.   d. stratum spinosum.   ____

81. The least severe skin cancer is:
    a. basal cell carcinoma.
    b. malignant melanoma.
    c. basal cell melanoma.
    d. squamous cell carcinoma. ____

82. Acquired canities is the result of:
    a. previous over-processing.   c. poor nutrition.
    b. a fungus.   d. genetics. ____

83. Hair that has a hard, glassy finish is:
    a. wiry.   c. coarse.
    b. fine.   d. medium. ____

84. The pH range for hair conditioners is:
    a. 4.5 to 7.5.   c. 3.0 to 5.5.
    b. 2.0 to 4.5.   d. 6.0 to 8.5. ____

85. The color of the skin depends on genetics and:
    a. keratin.   c. melanin.
    b. collagen.   d. sebum. ____

86. A condition of abnormal hair growth is:
    a. trichoptilosis.   c. trichorrhexis nodosa.
    b. hypertrichosis.   d. canities. ____

87. The degree of coarseness or fineness of individual hair
    strands is hair:
    a. elasticity.   c. texture.
    b. density.   d. porosity. ____

88. A chronic bacterial infection surrounding the follicles of the
    beard and mustache areas is called:
    a. pseudofolliculitis barbae.   c. folliculitis barbae.
    b. a furuncle.   d. sycosis vulgaris. ____

89. A conditioner that can weigh down fine hair, leaving it flat or
    oily, is:
    a. spray-on.   c. cuticle-coating.
    b. light leave-in.   d. scalp. ____

90. Dermatitis lesions may appear as:
    a. nodules.   c. vesicles.
    b. wheals.   d. fissures. ____

91. Oily scalp and hair is caused by:
- **a.** poor blood circulation to the scalp.
- **b.** overactive sebaceous glands.
- **c.** inactivity of the oil glands.
- **d.** the fungus ma lassezia.   ____

92. Tinea barbae is a superficial fungal infection occurring over the:
- **a.** entire scalp.
- **c.** nape of the neckline.
- **b.** bearded area of the face.
- **d.** top of the scalp.   ____

93. The term used to describe abnormal hair loss is:
- **a.** malassezia.
- **c.** dandruff.
- **b.** alopecia.
- **d.** pediculosis capitis.   ____

94. Eyebrow hairs and eyelashes are replaced every:
- **a.** 75 to 100 days.
- **c.** 6 months.
- **b.** 1 to 2 months.
- **d.** 4 to 5 months.   ____

95. A birthmark is also known as a:
- **a.** chloasma.
- **c.** vitiligo.
- **b.** nevus.
- **d.** stain.   ____

96. The cycle of hair growth where new hair is grown is:
- **a.** anagen.
- **c.** androgen.
- **b.** catagen.
- **d.** telogen.   ____

97. An example of a chemical modality is:
- **a.** microcurrent.
- **c.** microdermabrasion.
- **b.** lasers.
- **d.** galvanic.   ____

98. A tuft of hair that stands straight up is a:
- **a.** cowlick.
- **c.** whorl.
- **b.** hair stream.
- **d.** vellus.   ____

99. A characteristic of scabies is:
- **a.** excessive itching.
- **b.** brittle hair.
- **c.** dry, sulfur-yellow, cuplike crusts.
- **d.** musty odor.   ____

100. Skin tags most frequently occur on the:
- **a.** scalp.
- **c.** hands and feet.
- **b.** neck and chest.
- **d.** face.   ____

101. The tendon that connects the occipitalis and frontalis is the:
- **a.** procerus.
- **b.** epicranial aponeurosis.
- **c.** epicranius.
- **d.** corrugator.

____

102. A stroking movement is used in:
- **a.** friction.
- **b.** percussion.
- **c.** effleurage.
- **d.** pétrissage.

____

103. An example of mechanical exfoliation is:
- **a.** steaming.
- **b.** direct surface application.
- **c.** brushing.
- **d.** desincrustation.

____

104. A positive electrode is a(n):
- **a.** anode.
- **b.** wavelength.
- **c.** cathode.
- **d.** high-frequency current.

____

105. Ultraviolet lamps treat:
- **a.** aging skin.
- **b.** wrinkles.
- **c.** dandruff.
- **d.** nerve disorders.

____

106. The muscle that bends and rotates the head is the:
- **a.** trapezius.
- **b.** platysma.
- **c.** sternocleidomastoideus.
- **d.** zygomaticus minor.

____

107. The most stimulating form of massage is:
- **a.** effleurage.
- **b.** percussion.
- **c.** pétrissage.
- **d.** friction.

____

108. The products that work best for combination skin types are:
- **a.** oil-based.
- **b.** water-oil-based.
- **c.** water-based.
- **d.** alcohol-based.

____

109. Hairline shapes are determined by:
- **a.** hair texture.
- **b.** facial-hair design.
- **c.** skin type.
- **d.** growth patterns.

____

110. Ingrown hairs are called:
- **a.** folliculitis.
- **b.** a keloid condition.
- **c.** pseudofolliculitis.
- **d.** pustules.

____

111. An example of an electric current modality is:
- **a.** an electric massager.
- **b.** lasers.
- **c.** high frequency.
- **d.** infrared devices.

____

112. An example of a chemical exfoliant is a(n):
   a. enzyme peel.
   c. emollient.
   b. astringent.
   d. granular scrub. ____

113. The way the razor is held in the barber's hand to perform a stroke movement is referred to as the:
   a. grain.
   c. position.
   b. procedure.
   d. angle. ____

114. An example of an antihemorrhagic is:
   a. astringent.
   b. pH-balanced fresheners or toners.
   c. styptic powder.
   d. alcohol. ____

115. Toners:
   a. remove dead cells from the skin surface.
   b. add moisture to the skin surface.
   c. tighten the skin.
   d. draw impurities out of pores. ____

116. The chief sensory nerve of the face is the:
   a. eleventh cranial.
   c. facial.
   b. seventh cranial.
   d. fifth cranial. ____

117. The razor position and stroke *not* used in facial shaving is the:
   a. backhand.
   c. reverse freehand.
   b. reverse backhand.
   d. freehand. ____

118. The average rate of hair growth per month is:
   a. 1½ inches.
   c. ¼ inch.
   b. I inch.
   d. ½ inch. ____

119. The facial shape that has over-wide cheekbones and a narrow jaw line is the:
   a. inverted triangular.
   c. oval.
   b. diamond.
   d. pear-shaped. ____

120. A type of mask that employs the pack application method is:
   a. clay.
   c. gel.
   b. paraffin wax.
   d. cream. ____

121. The massage movement that stimulates the nerves to tone the muscles is:
   a. pétrissage.
   c. percussion.
   b. friction.
   d. effleurage. ____

122. Skin that allows the beard hair to be cut more easily is:
- **a.** taut.
- **c.** loose.
- **b.** dry.
- **d.** tight. _____

123. The facial shape recognized as the ideal shape is:
- **a.** square.
- **c.** oblong.
- **b.** round.
- **d.** oval. _____

124. The type of beard that would help to fill out a narrow jaw is:
- **a.** full.
- **c.** rounded.
- **b.** square.
- **d.** close-cut. _____

125. Finishing a shave includes:
- **a.** stretching the skin.
- **b.** massaging moisturizer into the skin.
- **c.** lathering the face with cream or gel.
- **d.** steaming the face. _____

126. The profile that has a prominent forehead and chin is:
- **a.** concave.
- **c.** straight.
- **b.** angular.
- **d.** convex. _____

127. An important design element when discussing balance is hair:
- **a.** color.
- **c.** density.
- **b.** porosity.
- **d.** texture. _____

128. A variation of the taper cutis the:
- **a.** brush cut.
- **c.** quo vadis cut.
- **b.** businessman's cut.
- **d.** butch cut. _____

129. The most popular hair choice when it comes to hair replacement is:
- **a.** human.
- **c.** chemically treated.
- **b.** synthetic.
- **d.** mixed. _____

130. You should discard used blades in a:
- **a.** closed receptacle.
- **c.** sharps container.
- **b.** plastic garbage bag.
- **d.** trash basket. _____

131. The way the hair is attached to the base of the hair solution is called:
- **a.** root-turning.
- **c.** looping.
- **b.** fitting.
- **d.** knotting. _____

132. All the hair strands end at one level to form a heavy weight line at the perimeter in the:
- **a.** graduated cut.
- **b.** uniform-layered cut.
- **c.** blunt cut.
- **d.** long-layered cut.

_____

133. The most commonly used permrod is:
- **a.** bender.
- **b.** loop.
- **c.** concave.
- **d.** straight.

_____

134. Relaxers sold in base and no-base formulas are:
- **a.** chemical neutralizing.
- **b.** hydroxide.
- **c.** ammonium thioglycolate.
- **d.** base neutralizing.

_____

135. While shaving, the skin should be:
- **a.** cold.
- **b.** moist.
- **c.** hot.
- **d.** dry.

_____

136. Ready-to-wear wigs are made of:
- **a.** a synthetic fiber.
- **b.** wool.
- **c.** angora.
- **d.** yak hair.

_____

137. The elevation for a graduated cut is:
- **a.** 180 degrees.
- **b.** 90 degrees.
- **c.** 0 degrees.
- **d.** 45 degrees.

_____

138. An ownership structure controlled by one or more stockholders is a:
- **a.** partnership.
- **b.** corporation.
- **c.** sole proprietorship.
- **d.** franchise.

_____

139. A salary-plus-commission compensation arrangement is a(n):
- **a.** default.
- **b.** guarantee.
- **c.** percentage.
- **d.** upsell.

_____

140. A series of connected dots that results in a continuous mark is a(n):
- **a.** shape.
- **b.** outline.
- **c.** form.
- **d.** line.

_____

141. The act of recommending and selling products to your clients for at-home use is:
- **a.** upselling.
- **b.** ticket upgrading.
- **c.** servicing.
- **d.** retailing.

_____

142. On the exam, the questions you should answer first are the:
- **a.** easiest ones.
- **b.** shortest ones.
- **c.** longest ones.
- **d.** difficult ones. _____

143. On your resume you should stress your:
- **a.** salary requirements.
- **b.** technological savvy.
- **c.** personal information.
- **d.** accomplishments. _____

144. The hair's ability to absorb haircoloring products is determined by:
- **a.** elasticity.
- **b.** texture.
- **c.** porosity.
- **d.** density. _____

145. The outer perimeter line of the haircut is the:
- **a.** cutting line.
- **b.** guideline.
- **c.** parting.
- **d.** design line. _____

146. The primary concern when constructing the best physical layout for a barbershop is:
- **a.** retail sales.
- **b.** costs.
- **c.** personnel.
- **d.** maximum efficiency. _____

147. An indication of the strength of the hair's cortex is:
- **a.** texture.
- **b.** elasticity.
- **c.** density.
- **d.** porosity. _____

148. A typical question asked on an interview would be:
- **a.** What is your native language?
- **b.** Are you a U.S. citizen?
- **c.** What skills do you feel are your strongest?
- **d.** How old are you? _____

149. A guide to the actions of the organization is a:
- **a.** mission statement.
- **b.** goal.
- **c.** business plan.
- **d.** vision statement. _____

150. A variation of the crew cut is the:
- **a.** flat top.
- **b.** Princeton cut.
- **c.** precision cut.
- **d.** brush cut. _____

SAMPLE STATE BOARD
EXAMINATION TEST 2

1. A written description of your business as you see it today and as you foresee it in the next 5 years is a:
   - **a.** written agreement.
   - **b.** brand identity.
   - **c.** business plan.
   - **d.** benchmark.
   _____

2. A key to teamwork is:
   - **a.** communication.
   - **b.** determination.
   - **c.** competition.
   - **d.** ambition.
   _____

3. Tips must be tracked and reported on your:
   - **a.** daily log.
   - **b.** income tax return.
   - **c.** monthly budget worksheet.
   - **d.** individual retirement account.
   _____

4. The basic question or problem is the:
   - **a.** choice.
   - **b.** statement.
   - **c.** stem.
   - **d.** key word.
   _____

5. During an interview, questions are permitted regarding:
   - **a.** medical conditions.
   - **b.** date of birth.
   - **c.** disabilities.
   - **d.** drug or tobacco use.
   _____

6. A state that does not allow booth rental is:
   - **a.** Pennsylvania.
   - **b.** New York.
   - **c.** Vermont.
   - **d.** South Dakota.
   _____

7. Reaching logical conclusions by employing logical reasoning is:
   - **a.** objective reasoning.
   - **b.** relative reasoning.
   - **c.** deductive reasoning.
   - **d.** effective reasoning.
   _____

8. The least expensive way of owning your own business is a:
   - **a.** independent local chain.
   - **b.** spa.
   - **c.** regional franchise shop.
   - **d.** booth rental.
   _____

9. A reduction in the production of melanin pigments results in:
   - **a.** white hair.
   - **b.** dark blond hair.
   - **c.** light blond hair.
   - **d.** gray hair.
   _____

10. The type of lighting not suitable for judging existing haircolors is:
    a. a well-lit room.   c. incandescent.
    b. strong natural light.   d. fluorescent.   _____

11. The first goal of every business is to:
    a. upsell your clients.
    b. add more services.
    c. sell retail products.
    d. maintain current clients.   _____

12. The words you should look for in true/false questions are:
    a. related words.   c. similar words.
    b. qualifying words.   d. absolute words.   _____

13. You should follow up an interview with a:
    a. request for a job offer.
    b. thank-you gift.
    c. thank-you note.
    d. request for a second interview. _____

14. White hair is the color of keratin without:
    a. eumelanin.   c. base color.
    b. pheomelanin.   d. melanin.   _____

15. The process of coloring hair back to its natural color is:
    a. retouching.
    b. a tint back.
    c. pre-softening.
    d. single-process haircoloring.   _____

16. When the employer pays you solely through a percentage of the gross service sales you generate, you are being compensated as:
    a. salary-plus-commission.   c. straight salary.
    b. hourly salary.   d. commission.   _____

17. An example of a warm color is:
    a. green.   c. blue.
    b. violet.   d. red.   _____

18. Lighteners that add temporary color as they lighten are called:
    a. quick lighteners.   c. powder lighteners.
    b. neutral oil lighteners.   d. color oil lighteners. _____

19. A Jheri® curl is also known as:
    a. permanent waving.   c. curl reformation.
    b. chemical waving.   d. chemical hair relaxing. _____

20. Hair that has a raised cuticle layer that easily absorbs chemical solutions is:
    a. resistant.
    c. dense.
    b. coarse.
    d. porous.
    _____

21. Not paying back your loans is:
    a. defaulting.
    c. charging.
    b. forgiving.
    d. borrowing.
    _____

22. The warmth or coolness of a color is:
    a. hue.
    c. natural level.
    b. intensity.
    d. tone.
    _____

23. To correct excessive porosity, you would use:
    a. toners.
    c. solvents.
    b. fillers.
    d. removers.
    _____

24. The layer that provides strength, elasticity, and natural color to the hair is the:
    a. cuticle.
    c. protein.
    b. cortex.
    d. medulla.
    _____

25. The wrap that uses one paper folded in half over the ends of the hair is the:
    a. bookend wrap.
    c. double flat wrap.
    b. single flat wrap.
    d. double-end wrap.
    _____

26. When you are committed to consistently doing a good job for your clients, employer, and barbershop team you have:
    a. integrity.
    c. good technical skills.
    b. a strong work ethic.
    d. motivation.
    _____

27. A demipermanent color:
    a. creates fun, bold results that easily shampoo from the hair.
    b. acts as a filler in color correction.
    c. neutralizes yellow or other unwanted tones.
    d. adds subtle color results.
    _____

28. Hair that may be more resistant to chemical processes is:
    a. fine.
    c. coarse.
    b. porous.
    d. medium.
    _____

29. Rods used when a definite wave pattern, close to the head, is desired are:
    a. circle tool rods.
    c. straight rods.
    b. bender rods.
    d. concave rods.
    _____

30. The main oxidizing agent used in haircoloring is:
- **a.** hydrogen peroxide.
- **b.** metallic salts.
- **c.** aniline derivatives.
- **d.** bleach. ____

31. The three primary colors are red, blue, and:
- **a.** white.
- **b.** gray.
- **c.** yellow.
- **d.** black. ____

32. The rod that creates a consistently sized wave from one side of the hair parting to the other is the:
- **a.** loop rod.
- **b.** straight rod.
- **c.** concave rod.
- **d.** bender rod. ____

33. The reducing agent in alkaline perms is:
- **a.** glyceryl monothioglycolate.
- **b.** alkanolamines.
- **c.** ammonium thioglycolate.
- **d.** hydrogen peroxide. ____

34. The oldest and most commonly used chemical relaxer is:
- **a.** lithium hydroxide.
- **b.** sodium hydroxide.
- **c.** thio.
- **d.** guanidine hydroxide. ____

35. Thick, coarse hair types are easier to cut with:
- **a.** clippers.
- **b.** scissors.
- **c.** shears.
- **d.** razors. ____

36. Another term for an activator is:
- **a.** accelerator.
- **b.** generator.
- **c.** developer.
- **d.** lightener. ____

37. Perm wraps begin with sectioning the hair into:
- **a.** bands.
- **b.** contours.
- **c.** panels.
- **d.** patterns. ____

38. Thinning the hair to graduated lengths with the shears is:
- **a.** carving.
- **b.** texturing.
- **c.** slicing.
- **d.** slithering. ____

39. The part of the curl that is between the scalp and the first arc of the circle is the:
- **a.** foundation.
- **b.** base.
- **c.** barrel.
- **d.** stem. ____

40. The perm pattern that blends hair from one area to another is the:
- **a.** bricklay.
- **b.** piggyback.
- **c.** basic.
- **d.** curvature. ____

41. One of the most important characteristics when choosing haircolor tint shades is:
    a. density.   c. texture.
    b. porosity.   d. elasticity.   _____

42. Once a graduated haircut is dry, you should:
    a. comb the hair to natural fall.
    b. detangle the hair with the wide-tooth comb.
    c. detail the perimeter.
    d. texturize the interior.   _____

43. The best evidence of pleased and satisfied clients is/are:
    a. personal referrals.   c. increased advertising.
    b. social media marketing.   d. a network fan page. _____

44. The haircutting technique that blends short and long lengths along a perimeter design line or interior section is:
    a. overdirection.   c. razor cutting.
    b. notching.   d. texturizing.   _____

45. One of the benefits of alkaline perms are:
    a. strong curl patterns.
    b. slower, but more controllable processing times.
    c. gentler treatments for delicate hair types.
    d. softer curl patterns.   _____

46. For coloring mustaches, you should never use:
    a. pomades.   c. aniline derivative tints.
    b. liquid tints.   d. hair color crayons. _____

47. Rods used for a spiral wrap are:
    a. circlerods.   c. straight rods.
    b. loop rods.   d. concave rods.   _____

48. The position of the wave rod or tool in relation to its base section is the:
    a. base direction.   c. base control.
    b. wrapping pattern.   d. wave formation.   _____

49. Strong alkalis that can swell the hair up to twice its normal diameter are:
    a. neutralizers.   c. thio relaxers.
    b. waving solutions.   d. hydroxide relaxers. _____

50. Tones that indicate overlightening are:
    a. ash.   c. violet.
    b. gold.   d. red.   _____

51. For the uniform-layered cut, you should dry the hair:
    a   With a round brush.   c. with a diffuser.
    b. with your hands.   d. naturally.   ____

52. Hair products used in the manufacture of theatrical or fashion wigs are:
    a. synthetic.   c. chemically treated.
    b. mixed.   d. human.   ____

53. Re-conditioning treatments should be given to prevent hair replacement systems from:
    a. fading.   c. brittleness.
    b. matting.   d. yellowing.   ____

54. The widest section of the head is the:
    a. four corners.   c. occipital bone.
    b. parietal ridge.   d. apex.   ____

55. To create design lines at the perimeter of the haircut, the technique you would use is:
    a. freehand shear cutting.
    b. cutting palm-to-palm.
    c. cutting below the fingers.
    d. cutting above the fingers.   ____

56. The hair solution recommended when the hair is worn in an off-the-face style is:
    a. full-head bonding.   c. cover-up.
    b. partial lace fill-in.   d. lace-front.   ____

57. The parietal ridge is known as the:
    a. horseshoe.   c. apex.
    b. guideline.   d. projection.   ____

58. A medium to long taper cut with a long top section is a:
    a. classic pompadour.   c. quo vadis.
    b. classic Caesar.   d. butch cut.   ____

59. Before shaving the head, you should analyze the scalp to identify:
    a. hair growth patterns.   c. hypertrophies.
    b. the sections of the head.   d. hair density.   ____

60. A wet styling technique that shapes and directs the hair into an S pattern is:
    a. coiling.   c. finger waving.
    b. double twisting.   d. scrunch styling.   ____

61. The process of attaching a hair replacement system to the head with an adhesive bonding agent is known as:
    a. a partial hair solution.   c. lace-front.
    b. full-head bonding.   d. partial lace fill-in.   ____

62. Hairstyles that are tapered slightly higher to above the occipital are:
    a. medium-length.   c. longer.
    b. fade.   d. semi-short.   ____

63. The cutting technique freehand slicing is also known as:
    a. razor rotation.   c. freehand clipper.
    b. razor-over-comb.   d. fingers-and-razor.   ____

64. Whenever not in use, a razor should be:
    a. in a sharps container.   c. empty of a blade.
    b. closed.   d. open.   ____

65. You should not proceed with the shave service if the client has:
    a. pustules.   c. ingrown hairs.
    b. a keloid condition.   d. chapped skin.   ____

66. Synthetic hair solutions should be cleaned with:
    a. cold water.   c. hot water.
    b. re-conditioners.   d. a solvent.   ____

67. Most men's haircuts require some form of:
    a. thinning.   c. texturing.
    b. layering.   d. tapering.   ____

68. The result of improper hair removal by a razor, tweezers, or trimmer are:
    a. whorls.   c. ingrown hairs.
    b. pustules.   d. skin infections.   ____

69. The shaving movement from the angle of the mouth towards the point of the chin is:
    a. reverse freehand and up.   c. freehand and across.
    b. backhand and down.   d. freehand and down.   ____

70. The shave that should result in a smooth face without being a close shave is the:
    a. second-time-over.   c. first-time-over.
    b. outline.   d. once-over.   ____

71. To blend the ends of are placement with the client's natural hair you use:
    a. a razor.
    b. clippers.
    c. haircutting shears.
    d. thinning shears. ____

72. The heaviest perimeter area of a 0-elevation or 45-degree cut is the:
    a. weight line.
    b. horizontal line.
    c. cutting line.
    d. vertical line. ____

73. The most popular technique for eyebrow trimming is:
    a. razor cutting.
    b. clipper-over-comb.
    c. cutting below the fingers.
    d. shear-over-comb. ____

74. You should not use hot towels on skin that is:
    a. freckled.
    b. chapped.
    c. tanned.
    d. wrinkled. ____

75. The shaving strokes you use around the mouth, over the ears, and in other tight areas are:
    a. medium.
    b. shorter.
    c. faster.
    d. longer. ____

76. The mustache that would be complimentary for a man with an extra-large mouth is:
    a. medium to large.
    b. pyramid-shaped.
    c. heavier-looking.
    d. semi-square. ____

77. An example of a heat modality is:
    a. low-level laser therapy.
    b. microcurrents.
    c. low-level light therapy.
    d. infrared devices. ____

78. The muscle that covers the back of the neck allowing movement of the shoulders is the:
    a. sternocleidomastoideus.
    b. trapezius.
    c. triangularis.
    d. platysma. ____

79. The vessels that transport oxygenated blood from the heart to all parts of the body are:
    a. veins.
    b. arteries.
    c. capillaries.
    d. venules. ____

80. The gentlest form of tapotement is:
    a. tapping.
    b. kneading.
    c. stroking.
    d. hacking. ____

81. The correct angle of cutting with a razor is called the:
- **a.** cutting stroke.
- **c.** freehand stroke.
- **b.** proper stroke.
- **d.** gliding stroke.

_____

82. The broad muscle that covers the top of the skull is the:
- **a.** epicranius.
- **c.** occipitalis.
- **b.** epicranial aponeurosis.
- **d.** frontalis.

_____

83. The massage movement that exerts an invigorating effect on the area being massaged is:
- **a.** percussion.
- **c.** effleurage.
- **b.** tapotement.
- **d.** pétrissage.

_____

84. The use of an anode to introduce an acid-pH product into the skin is:
- **a.** cataphoresis.
- **c.** desincrustation.
- **b.** high-frequency.
- **d.** anaphoresis.

_____

85. Shampoos are:
- **a.** creams.
- **c.** solvents.
- **b.** emulsions.
- **d.** ointments.

_____

86. Shaving preparation includes:
- **a.** toning.
- **b.** massaging moisturizer into the skin.
- **c.** draping the client.
- **d.** light powder dusting.

_____

87. One of the muscle groups that coordinate opening and closing the mouth are the:
- **a.** mentalis.
- **c.** buccinators.
- **b.** risorius.
- **d.** masseter.

_____

88. The massage manipulation that has proven to be beneficial to the circulation and glandular activity of the skin is:
- **a.** friction.
- **c.** tapotement.
- **b.** vibration.
- **d.** percussion.

_____

89. To treat surface wrinkles and aging skin you could use:
- **a.** anaphoresis.
- **c.** light therapy.
- **b.** microdermabrasion.
- **d.** cataphoresis.

_____

90. All of the following characteristics of hair should be considered before choosing products except:
- **a.** hair density.
- **c.** hair length.
- **b.** hair porosity.
- **d.** hair texture.

_____

91. The shave that should ensure a complete and even shave with a single lathering is the:
    a. second-time-over.   c. once-over.
    b. close.   d. first-time-over.   ____

92. The muscle you use when laughing is the:
    a. zygomaticus major.   c. mentalis.
    b. triangularis.   d. orbicularis oris.   ____

93. The galvanic treatment that uses a very low level of electrical current for applications in skin care is:
    a. microcurrent.   c. desincrustation.
    b. iontophoresis.   d. microdermabrasion.   ____

94. An effective way to prepare the scalp for scalp massage manipulations and treatments is a(n):
    a. hand massager.   c. scalp steam.
    b. electric massager.   d. hair tonic.   ____

95. The tube-like depression or pocket in the skin or scalp that contains the hair root is the:
    a. dermal papilla.   c. hair bulb.
    b. hair follicle.   d. arrector pili.   ____

96. The most successful cutting technique for beards with even density and texture is:
    a. shear-over-comb.   c. outliner-over-comb.
    b. razor cutting.   d. even-all-over clipper.   ____

97. The motor nerve that controls motions of the neck and shoulder muscles is the:
    a. trifacial nerve.   c. fifth cranial nerve.
    b. accessory nerve.   d. seventh cranial nerve.   ____

98. The skin treatment that can assist the body in producing vitamin D is/are:
    a. ultraviolet lamps.   c. microcurrents.
    b. microdermabrasion.   d. infrared rays.   ____

99. Hair that may require a humectant-rich moisturizing conditioner to increase manageability is:
    a. fine, brittle hair.   c. chemically treated hair.
    b. dry, coarse hair.   d. oily hair.   ____

100. To relieve pain in sore muscles you could use:
    a. ultraviolet rays.   c. desincrustation.
    b. infrared rays.   d. high-frequency current.   ____

101. The structure that contains the blood and nerve supply that provides the nutrients needed for hair growth is in the:
   a. dermal papilla.
   c. medulla.
   b. arrector pili.
   d. cortex. _____

102. Hair that has low elasticity, breaks easily, and has a tendency to knot, especially on the ends, is:
   a. extremely curly.
   c. extremely straight.
   b. wavy.
   d. curly. _____

103. The alopecia also known as male pattern baldness is:
   a. alopecia prematura.
   c. androgenic alopecia.
   b. alopecia senilis.
   d. alopecia universalis. _____

104. The layer of the skin responsible for the growth of the epidermis is:
   a. stratum germinativum.
   c. stratum corneum.
   b. stratum spinosum.
   d. stratum granulosum. _____

105. A disorder of the sebaceous glands associated with newborn babies is:
   a. whiteheads.
   c. seborrhea.
   b. milia.
   d. open comedo. _____

106. The layer of hair that may be absent in very fine and naturally blond hair is the:
   a. medulla.
   c. keratin.
   b. cuticle.
   d. cortex. _____

107. A sensitive topic that you can speak to your client about is:
   a. marital problems.
   b. mental health concerns.
   c. money problems.
   d. abnormal hair loss. _____

108. Subcutaneous tissue is also known as:
   a. connective tissue.
   c. adipose tissue.
   b. fibrous tissue.
   d. elastic tissue. _____

109. An absence of melanin pigment in the body is known as:
   a. albinism.
   c. chloasma.
   b. hyperpigmentation.
   d. leukoderma. _____

110. Hair with a high porosity level Is usually the result of:
   a. internal disorders.
   b. poor nutrition.
   c. hormonal changes.
   d. previous over-processing. _____

111. Protein is made of:
    a. disulfides.
    b. hydroxides.
    c. amino acids.
    d. pH.   _____

112. A topical treatment proven to stimulate hair growth is:
    a. minoxidil.
    b. Propecia.
    c. finasteride.
    d. malassezia.   _____

113. The type of nerve fibers that carry impulses from the brain to the muscles are:
    a. secretory.
    b. receptor.
    c. motor.
    d. sensory.   _____

114. A function of the skin that protects the body from the environment is:
    a. excretion.
    b. heat regulation.
    c. absorption.
    d. secretion.   _____

115. Excessive oiliness on the skin or scalp may be:
    a. telangiectasis.
    b. rosacea.
    c. milia.
    d. seborrhea.   _____

116. Hair that is long, coarse, found on the scalp, legs, arms, and bodies of males and females is:
    a. medulla.
    b. lanugo.
    c. vellus.
    d. terminal.   _____

117. The term that is applied most frequently to a folliculit is barbae condition is:
    a. a boil.
    b. male pattern baldness.
    c. barber's itch.
    d. razor bumps.   _____

118. Loosening of the elastic skin fibers due to abnormal tension or relaxation of the facial muscles influences the formation of:
    a. wrinkles.
    b. goose bumps.
    c. skin tags.
    d. fatty tissue.   _____

119. If the hair that feels smooth and the cuticle is compact, it is considered:
    a. over processed.
    b. over-porous.
    c. porous.
    d. resistant.   _____

120. An abnormal mass varying in size, shape, and color is a:
    a. tumor.
    b. bulla.
    c. nodule.
    d. cyst.   _____

121. The hair growth phase where the follicle shrinks, the hair bulb disappears, and the shrunken root end forms a rounded club is:
    a. telogen.
    b. catagen.
    c. androgen.
    d. anagen.
    _____

122. An acute, deep-seated bacterial infection in the subcutaneous tissue results ina:
    a. carbuncle.
    b. furuncle.
    c. razor bump.
    d. boil.
    _____

123. One characteristic of aged skin is its:
    a. loss of color.
    b. formation of blackheads.
    c. oiliness.
    d. loss of elasticity.
    _____

124. The body system that controls the activity of sweat glands is the:
    a. endocrine.
    b. nervous system.
    c. circulatory.
    d. lymphatic/immune.
    _____

125. An example of a bulla is:
    a. impetigo.
    b. a liver spot.
    c. severe acne.
    d. lipoma.
    _____

126. Hair that is more susceptible to damage from chemical services is:
    a. wiry.
    b. fine.
    c. medium.
    d. coarse.
    _____

127. The skin protects the body from:
    a. emotional stress.
    b. pain.
    c. pathogens.
    d. pressure.
    _____

128. The flow of electricity along a conductor is a(n):
    a. electric circuit.
    b. rheostat.
    c. electric current.
    d. insulator.
    _____

129. The term that applies to all living things and those things that were once alive is:
    a. matter.
    b. element.
    c. organic.
    d. inorganic.
    _____

130. Shampoos that are mild formulations designed to prevent the stripping of haircolor from the hair are:
    a. pH-balanced.
    b. balancing.
    c. color-enhancing.
    d. clarifying.
    _____

131. An adjustable resistor used for controlling the current in a circuit is a(n):
  a. insulator.
  b. rectifier.
  c. rheostat.
  d. battery-operated instrument.   ____

132. An example of an instant conditioner is a:
  a. dandruff rinse.   **c.** detangling rinse.
  b. permanent wave product.   **d.** blowdrying spray.   ____

133. The study of the functions and activities performed by the body's structures is:
  a. histology.   **c.** osteology.
  b. physiology.   **d.** anatomy.   ____

134. The part of the cell that plays an important part in cell reproduction and metabolism is the:
  a. nucleus.   **c.** cytoplasm.
  b. cell membrane.   **d.** protoplasm.   ____

135. Organic chemistry is the study of substances that contain:
  a. hydrogen.   **c.** oxygen.
  b. sulfur.   **d.** carbon.   ____

136. When using an electrical appliance, you should not touch:
  a. plastic.   **c.** glass.
  b. rubber.   **d.** metal.   ____

137. The tissue that carries messages to and from the brain and controls and coordinates all bodily functions is:
  a. connective.   **c.** epithelial.
  b. muscle.   **d.** nerve.   ____

138. A comb that is antistatic is made from:
  a. hard rubber.   **c.** carbon materials.
  b. graphite.   **d.** metal.   ____

139. The agency that registers all types of disinfectants sold and used in the United States is:
  a. OSHA.   **c.** the CDC.
  b. the U.S. Department of Labor.   **d.** the EPA.   ____

140. The first step in good hygiene is:
  a. not smoking during work hours.
  b. using mouthwash.
  c. hand washing.
  d. brushing your teeth.   ____

141. The light rays used in ultraviolet germicidal irradiation to inactivate or destroy microorganisms are:
- **a.** infrared light.
- **b.** visible light.
- **c.** UVC rays.
- **d.** UVB rays. _____

142. An example of a pure substance is:
- **a.** concrete.
- **b.** aluminum foil.
- **c.** salt water solution.
- **d.** powder. _____

143. When standing, your spine should be:
- **a.** relaxed.
- **b.** slightly curved.
- **c.** elongated.
- **d.** straight. _____

144. An example of emulsions used in barbering services are:
- **a.** soaps.
- **b.** conditioners.
- **c.** powders.
- **d.** hair tonics. _____

145. An electric clipper with a pivot motor would be used to cut:
- **a.** thick, coarse, or damp hair.
- **b.** dry and fine hair.
- **c.** thick and dry hair.
- **d.** all types of hair. _____

146. When using LEDs, the color light that reduces acne and bacteria is:
- **a.** blue.
- **b.** yellow.
- **c.** red.
- **d.** green. _____

147. An example of a physical change is:
- **a.** oxidation.
- **b.** ice melting to water.
- **c.** burning wood.
- **d.** rusting iron. _____

148. The bone that joins all of the bones of the cranium together is the:
- **a.** temporal.
- **b.** ethmoid.
- **c.** sphenoid.
- **d.** parietal. _____

149. A pH below 7 indicates a(n):
- **a.** alkaline solution.
- **b.** neutral solution.
- **c.** acidic solution.
- **d.** logarithmic solution. _____

150. A chemical compound that can exist in all three states of matter depending on its temperature is:
- **a.** hydrogen.
- **b.** oxygen.
- **c.** water.
- **d.** carbon dioxide. _____

SAMPLE STATE BOARD EXAMINATION TEST 3

1. The implements used during the glacial age for haircutting and styling were made of:
   - **a.** oyster shells.
   - **b.** copper.
   - **c.** iron.
   - **d.** ceramic. _____

2. Your outward appearance and conduct in the workplace projects your professional:
   - **a.** health.
   - **b.** image.
   - **c.** attitude.
   - **d.** success. _____

3. Bacteria that are harmful microorganisms and can cause disease or infection in humans are:
   - **a.** parasitic.
   - **b.** pathogenic.
   - **c.** infectious.
   - **d.** nonpathogenic. _____

4. You can irritate your lungs if you inhale the fumes from:
   - **a.** bleach.
   - **b.** detergents.
   - **c.** antiseptics.
   - **d.** alcohol. _____

5. The study of human body structures and how the body parts are organized is:
   - **a.** myology.
   - **b.** physiology.
   - **c.** histology.
   - **d.** anatomy. _____

6. During the Middle Ages, clergymen wore a distinguishing hair style known as a:
   - **a.** tonsure.
   - **b.** queue.
   - **c.** mustache.
   - **d.** wig. _____

7. To prevent fatigue and other physical problems, you should practice:
   - **a.** good posture.
   - **b.** repetitive motions.
   - **c.** physical therapies.
   - **d.** movement therapies. _____

8. Pus-forming bacteria that grow in clusters like bunches of grapes are:
   - **a.** streptococci.
   - **b.** cocci.
   - **c.** staphylococci.
   - **d.** diplococci. _____

9. You should remove hair particles from clipper blades with a:
   a. tong.
   b. scrub brush.
   c. nail brush.
   d. stiff brush.
   _____

10. The colorless jellylike substance found inside cells is:
    a. plasm.
    b. centrioles.
    c. cytoplasm.
    d. protoplasm.
    _____

11. The historical figure that encouraged shaving by imposing a tax on beards was:
    a. Emperor Hadrian.
    b. Peter the Great.
    c. Alexander the Great.
    d. Louis XIV.
    _____

12. The type of motion that can have a cumulative effect on muscles and joints is:
    a. steady.
    b. repetitive.
    c. downward.
    d. upward.
    _____

13. A fungicidal disinfectant is one capable of destroying:
    a. bacteria.
    b. parasites.
    c. viruses.
    d. molds.
    _____

14. Poisonous substances produced by some microorganisms, such as bacteria and viruses, are:
    a. pathogens.
    b. antitoxins.
    c. allergens.
    d. toxins.
    _____

15. An example of connective tissue is:
    a. the spinal cord.
    b. mucous membranes.
    c. blood.
    d. tissue inside the mouth.
    _____

16. The organization that develops standards for licensing and policing the barber industry is the:
    a. Associated Master Barbers and Beauticians of America.
    b. Barbers' Protective Association.
    c. National Association of Barber Boards of America.
    d. Journeymen Barbers International Union of America.
    _____

17. To avoid ergonomic-related injuries, the position your wrists should be held is:
    a. straight or neutral.
    b. erect.
    c. elongated and balanced.
    d. parallel to the floor.
    _____

18. Scrubbing using soap and water or detergent and water is considered:
a. disinfecting.   c. cleaning.
b. sanitizing.   d. sterilizing.   ____

19. The most common way a contagious infection is spread is/are:
a. water.   c. inhalation.
b. intact skin.   d. dirty hands.   ____

20. Body tissues are made up of large amounts of:
a. minerals.   c. nutrients.
b. water.   d. fat.   ____

21. An improvement to barbering over the past century has been:
a. educational standards.
b. relaxation of hygiene practices.
c. restriction of implement types.
d. the study of psychology.   ____

22. The key to avoiding musculoskeletal disorders in the barbering profession is:
a. movement therapy.   c. physical therapy.
b. a stress-free environment.   d. prevention.   ____

23. A single-celled microorganism with both plant and animal characteristics is a:
a. virus.   c. bacterium.
b. parasite.   d. fungus.   ____

24. The body prevents and controls infections through:
a. antitoxins.   c. red blood cells.
b. compromised skin.   d. uncompromised skin.   ____

25. Tissues that give smoothness and contour to the body are:
a. epithelial tissue.   c. nerve tissue.
b. muscle tissue.   d. adipose tissue.   ____

26. The time period that represented the heyday for American barbershops was the:
a. 1960s.   c. 1980s and 1990s.
b. 1940s and 1950s.   d. 1970s.   ____

27. An important human relations skill for a barber is:
a. attitude.   c. communication.
b. emotion.   d. education.   ____

28. A bloodborne virus that can live on a surface outside the body for long periods of time is:
- **a.** AIDS.
- **b.** HIV.
- **c.** hepatitis.
- **d.** tinea barbae.   ____

29. The type of electric clipper motor where the blades pull in one direction is the:
- **a.** universal motor.
- **b.** rotary motor.
- **c.** pivot motor.
- **d.** magnetic motor.   ____

30. Muscles found in the internal organs of the body are:
- **a.** striped.
- **b.** voluntary.
- **c.** nonstriated.
- **d.** striated.   ____

31. The red, white, and blue barber pole colors represent:
- **a.** haircutting, shaving, beard grooming.
- **b.** blood, veins, bandages.
- **c.** leeches, shaving cream, razors.
- **d.** life, water, porcelain.   ____

32. The interactions and relationships between two or more people is collectively called:
- **a.** communication.
- **b.** rapport.
- **c.** human relations.
- **d.** empathy.   ____

33. AIDS breaks down the body's:
- **a.** immune system.
- **b.** cardiovascular system.
- **c.** nervous system.
- **d.** endocrine system.   ____

34. Clipper blades are made of high-quality carbon steel or:
- **a.** plastic.
- **b.** ceramic.
- **c.** hard rubber.
- **d.** graphite.   ____

35. The muscles of the mouth that are used for grinning are the:
- **a.** mentalis muscles.
- **b.** risorius muscles.
- **c.** buccinator muscles.
- **d.** triangularis muscles.   ____

36. The settlers that brought barber-surgeons to America were the:
- **a.** French.
- **b.** Dutch and Swedish.
- **c.** Italians.
- **d.** Egyptians and Greeks.   ____

37. As a barber, you should be most concerned with the client's personal:
- **a.** grooming.
- **b.** hygiene habits.
- **c.** preferences.
- **d.** life.   ____

38. Effective sterilization requires the use of a(n):
    a. heat lamp.
    b. UV-ray cabinet.
    c. countertop receptacle.
    d. autoclave. _____

39. The razor of choice for professional barbering is the:
    a. safety razor.
    b. straight razor.
    c. edger.
    d. trimmer. _____

40. An example of an immovable joint is the:
    a. skull.
    b. knee.
    c. elbow.
    d. hip. _____

41. A time management tool that helps you to prioritize tasks and activities is:
    a. downtime.
    b. physical activity.
    c. unstructured time.
    d. a to-do list. _____

42. Specific standards of conduct that can be changed or updated frequently are:
    a. statues.
    b. regulations.
    c. laws.
    d. rules. _____

43. A form of formaldehyde that has a very high pH, and can damage the skin and eyes, are:
    a. bleaches.
    b. quaternary ammonium compounds.
    c. petroleum distillates.
    d. phenolic disinfectants. _____

44. The method for loose hair removal deemed no longer safe and sanitary is the:
    a. paper towel.
    b. neck duster.
    c. vacuum system.
    d. paper neck strip. _____

45. Painful inflammation of the wrist area can be caused by:
    a. keeping the wrist straight.
    b. prolonged standing.
    c. heat.
    d. repetitive motions. _____

46. The hours of sleep recommended by medical professionals are:
    a. 8 to 9.
    b. 7 to 8.
    c. 6 to 7.
    d. 5 to 6. _____

47. Disinfection is not effective against:
    a. bacteria spores.
    b. molds.
    c. viruses.
    d. bacteria. _____

48. Examples of known carcinogens are:
    a. bleaches.
    c. phenolics.
    b. distillates.
    d. quats.
    ____

49. The towel you use for a towel wrap should be:
    a. the neck duster.
    b. the styling towel.
    c. pre-steamed.
    d. 100 percent cotton terry cloth.
    ____

50. The body system that helps regulate the body's temperature is the:
    a. nervous system.
    b. circulatory system.
    c. integumentary system.
    d. lymphatic/immune system.
    ____

51. The negative or positive pole of an electric current is indicated by:
    a. modality.
    c. elasticity.
    b. polarity.
    d. activity.
    ____

52. The outermost hair layer is the:
    a. cortex.
    c. cuticle.
    b. medulla.
    d. follicle.
    ____

53. The immediate effect of massage is first noticed:
    a. in the muscles.
    b. In the hair follicles.
    c. through blood circulation.
    d. on the skin.
    ____

54. An insufficient flow of sebum from the sebaceous glands causes:
    a. combinations skin.
    c. normal skin.
    b. oily skin.
    d. dry skin.
    ____

55. The spleen is part of the:
    a. circulatory system.
    b. reproductive system.
    c. endocrine system.
    d. lymphatic/immune system.
    ____

56. One primary lesion that doesn't require a medical referral is:
    a. macule.
    c. papule.
    b. pustule.
    d. cyst.
    ____

57. Disulfide bonds can be broken by:
    a. pH.
    b. heat.
    c. chemical relaxers.
    d. water.   ____

58. To help soften follicle accumulation you should use:
    a. brushing.
    b. a galvanic machine.
    c. steam.
    d. high-frequency current.   ____

59. Alipidic skin is known as:
    a. dry skin.
    b. combination skin.
    c. normal skin.
    d. oily skin.   ____

60. The nerve that supplies impulses to the upper part of the face is the:
    a. ophthalmic nerve.
    b. maxillary nerve.
    c. infratrochlear nerve.
    d. mandibular nerve.   ____

61. Severely cracked or chapped hands or lips are examples of:
    a. keloids.
    b. ulcers.
    c. fissures.
    d. crusts.   ____

62. Natural hair color is the result of:
    a. chemical cross bonds.
    b. COHNS elements.
    c. amino acids.
    d. melanin pigment.   ____

63. The primary actions of high-frequency current are thermal and:
    a. tonic.
    b. therapeutic.
    c. systematic.
    d. antiseptic.   ____

64. A standard procedure when preparing the beard for shaving is applying:
    a. astringents.
    b. toners.
    c. hot towels.
    d. fresheners.   ____

65. The body system that passes on genetic code from one generation to another is the:
    a. integumentary system.
    b. endocrine system.
    c. reproductive system.
    d. lymphatic/immune system.   ____

66. An excoriation might be caused by:
    a. psoriasis.
    b. a post-operative repair.
    c. chicken pox.
    d. nail biting.   ____

67. Natural hair wave patterns are due to:
    a. age.
    b. genetics.
    c. melanin pigment.
    d. hormonal changes.   ____

68. Skin tissue can be destroyed with overexposure to:
    a. astringent solutions.
    b. microcrystals.
    c. ultraviolet rays.
    d. alkaline-pH products.   ____

69. When shaving, stretching the skin too tightly can cause:
    a. ingrown hairs.
    b. nicks.
    c. irritation.
    d. cuts.   ____

70. The bones of the fingers are the:
    a. phalanges.
    b. temporal bones.
    c. parietal bones.
    d. metacarpals.   ____

71. A disorder of the sudoriferous glands that can be life threatening is:
    a. anhidrosis.
    b. miliaria rubra.
    c. bromhidrosis.
    d. hyperhidrosis.   ____

72. Dandruff is due to:
    a. an acute, deep-seated bacterial infection.
    b. a fungus called malassezia.
    c. genetics.
    d. an active inflammatory process.   ____

73. To heat and relax the skin without increasing overall body temperature you use:
    a. galvanic currents.
    b. infrared rays.
    c. microcurrents.
    d. ultraviolet rays.   ____

74. To stretch or hold the skin firmly during the shave you should keep your fingers:
    a. gloved.
    b. dry.
    c. moist.
    d. powdered.   ____

75. Blood vessels that bring nutrients to the cells and carry away waste materials are called:
    a. capillaries.
    b. arteries.
    c. arterioles.
    d. venules.   ____

76. Foul-smelling perspiration could be caused by:
    a. miliaria rubra.
    b. anhidrosis.
    c. bromhidrosis.
    d. hyperhidrosis.   ____

77. The number of hairs on the head varies with the hair's:
    a. porosity.   c. color.
    b. elasticity.   d. coarseness.   ____

78. To perform desincrustation, a solution is applied to the skin's surface that is:
    a. astringent.
    b. basic.
    c. ion-containing water-soluble.
    d. acid-based.   ____

79. To establish proportionate design lines and contours, you use:
    a. partings.   c. guides.
    b. reference points.   d. cutting lines.   ____

80. The type of muscle not duplicated anywhere else in the body is the:
    a. striped muscle.   c. striated muscle.
    b. cardiac muscle.   d. nonstriated muscle. ____

81. A change in the pigmentation of the skin, known as a liver spot in older adults, is called:
    a. leukoderma.   c. lentigines.
    b. nevus.   d. chloasma.   ____

82. Wet hair has a tendency to stick to:
    a. synthetic material.   c. terry cloth.
    b. vinyl capes.   d. nylon capes.   ____

83. To produce chemical and ionic reactions in the skin, you use:
    a. ultraviolet rays.   c. galvanic current.
    b. Tesla current.   d. high-frequency current. ____

84. The quality of a form's surface is called its:
    a. proportion.   c. trough.
    b. design texture.   d. weight line.   ____

85. When oxygen is combined with a substance, the substance is said to be:
    a. oxidized.   c. blended.
    b. united.   d. reduced.   ____

86. If the thickening of a callus grows inward, it becomes a:
    a. blemish.   c. corn.
    b. verruca.   d. wart.   ____

87. The shampooing method where the client bends his head forward over the shampoo bowl or sink is the:
   a. massage method.
   c. inclined method.
   b. draping method.
   d. reclined method.
   _____

88. The follicle size of oily skin is:
   a. deeper.
   c. smaller.
   b. rounder.
   d. larger.
   _____

89. The line used to create one-length, low elevation or blunt haircut designs is the:
   a. vertical line.
   c. diagonal line.
   b. curved line.
   d. horizontal line.
   _____

90. Ingredients in wrinkle treatment creams are hormones and:
   a. glycerin.
   c. hydrolyzed protein.
   b. starch.
   d. collagen.
   _____

91. Eyes that are pink and skin that is sensitive to light are characteristics of:
   a. hyperpigmentation.
   c. vitiligo.
   b. albinism.
   d. lentigines.
   _____

92. The fifth cranial nerve is known as the:
   a. facial nerve.
   c. trigeminal nerve.
   b. cervical nerve.
   d. accessory nerve.
   _____

93. Cleansing creams:
   a. prevent moisture from evaporating.
   b. dissolve dirt and makeup.
   c. rebalance the pH of the skin.
   d. soften the skin.
   _____

94. Cutting the hair in the same direction in which it grows is called cutting:
   a. with a circular motion.
   c. against the grain.
   b. with the grain.
   d. across the grain.
   _____

95. To remove hair by pulling it out of the follicle you would use a(n):
   a. depilatory.
   c. epilator.
   b. mask.
   d. pack.
   _____

96. Sores that do not heal may be a symptom of:
   a. hypertrophies.
   b. dyschromias.
   c. skin cancer.
   d. disorders of the sudoriferous glands. ____

97. A beneficial result obtained by proper massage is:
   a. blood circulation is increased.
   b. nerves are aggravated.
   c. blood circulation is decreased.
   d. muscle fiber is reduced. ____

98. An example of an astringent is:
   a. witch hazel.   **c.** humectants.
   b. paraffin wax.   **d.** emollients. ____

99. The amount of tension used on straight hair to create precise lines is:
   a. minimum.   **c.** medium.
   b. maximum.   **d.** moderate. ____

100. The volt measures:
   a. electrical pressure.
   b. electrical resistance.
   c. strength or rate of electric current.
   d. amount of electric energy used in 1 second. ____

101. The cutting technique used for longer, tightly curled hair lengths that require more sculpting is:
   a. razor.   **c.** freehand shear.
   b. freehand clipper. **d.** clipper-over-comb. ____

102. The cut that will look soft and textured and conform to the head shape without weight lines or corners is the:
   a. graduated cut.   **c.** long-layered cut.
   b. uniform-layered cut. **d.** blunt cut. ____

103. A written summary of your education and work experience is a:
   a. template.   **c.** portfolio.
   b. resume.   **d.** cover letter. ____

104. Chemical reactions among proteins produce:
   a. peptide linkages.
   b. alkaline substances.
   c. glyceryl monothioglycolates.
   d. ammonium sulfites. ____

105. To replace ammonia, ammonia-free waves use:
- **a.** alkanolamines.
- **b.** cysteamines.
- **c.** bisulfites.
- **d.** mercaptamines.

_____

106. You would use a light stroke of the razor with very little pressure on:
- **a.** thick hair.
- **b.** fine hair.
- **c.** medium-textured hair.
- **d.** coarse hair.

_____

107. To set a pattern in the hair that will form the basis for a hairstyle you use:
- **a.** pin curls.
- **b.** curling irons.
- **c.** rollers.
- **d.** hair wraps.

_____

108. On your resume you should not state your:
- **a.** salary history.
- **b.** past accomplishments.
- **c.** professional references.
- **d.** skills mastered at other jobs.

_____

109. Cysteine is a(n):
- **a.** reducing agent.
- **b.** amino acid.
- **c.** alkali.
- **d.** oxidizing agent.

_____

110. A resistant strength of chemical waving products should be used on:
- **a.** porous hair.
- **b.** hair with less porosity.
- **c.** damaged hair.
- **d.** tinted hair.

_____

111. The cut where the top of the crest area looks squared off when viewed from the front is the:
- **a.** fade style.
- **b.** flat top.
- **c.** taper cut.
- **d.** precision cut.

_____

112. To perform a thermal waving you use:
- **a.** flat irons.
- **b.** heated pressing combs.
- **c.** Marcel irons.
- **d.** blowdryers.

_____

113. On your resume, begin accomplishment statements with:
- **a.** quallfying words.
- **b.** absolutes.
- **c.** action verbs.
- **d.** key words.

_____

114. The wrap used with short rods or short lengths of hair is the:
- **a.** single end wrap.
- **b.** double-end wrap.
- **c.** bookend wrap.
- **d.** double flat wrap.

_____

115. Texturizers and chemical blowouts are performed with a:
  a. guanidine hydroxide relaxer.
  b. lithium hydroxide relaxer.
  c. potassium hydroxide relaxer.
  d. thio relaxer. ____

116. The haircut that is cut with shears to create short, uniform layers is the:
  a. pompadour fade.
  b. flat top.
  c. classic Caesar.
  d. crew cut. ____

117. A guide to the actions of the organization that lays the foundation for how your company's strategies are created is called a(n):
  a. organizational plan.
  b. marketing plan.
  c. mission statement.
  d. vision statement. ____

118. A client consultation should take a(n):
  a. half hour.
  b. full appointment.
  c. few minutes.
  d. hour. ____

119. To smooth out the wrapping of uneven hair lengths, you use:
  a. fishhooks.
  b. relaxers.
  c. conditioners.
  d. end papers. ____

120. A chemical blowout removes some but not all:
  a. elasticity.
  b. curl.
  c. body.
  d. moisture. ____

121. For trimming excess hair in or around the ears, you could use:
  a. shears.
  b. an outliner.
  c. a straight razor.
  d. an electric razor. ____

122. Supplies used in daily business operation are:
  a. retail supplies.
  b. consumption supplies.
  c. merchandise supplies.
  d. service supplies. ____

123. If the elasticity is good, after stretching hair it will:
  a. tangle.
  b. curl.
  c. expand.
  d. contract. ____

124. Rods used for a body wave that serve as a foundation for further styling are:
  a. concave rods.
  b. large, straight rods.
  c. bender rods.
  d. circle tool rods. ____

125. Styling products used as part of the finishing process of a curl reformation are:

    a. moisturizers.
    c. texturizers.

    b. conditioners.
    d. pomades. _____

126. Popular for both men and women during the 1920s and 1930s was:

    a. scrunch styling.
    c. diffused drying.

    b. finger waving.
    d. braiding. _____

127. Most new shops begin operating at full capacity in:

    a. 3 months.
    c. 2 years.

    b. 6 months.
    d. 1 year. _____

128. The diameter of a single strand of hair is the measure of hair:

    a. texture.
    c. porosity.

    b. elasticity.
    d. density. _____

129. Half off-base rod placement results in:

    a. the least amount of volume.

    b. medium movement.

    c. greater volume at the scalp area.

    d. maximum movement. _____

130. Wet hair that does not return to its original length when stretched has:

    a. low elasticity.
    c. high porosity.

    b. low porosity.
    d. normal elasticity. _____

131. During the eighteenth century, the front section of hair was called the:

    a. club.
    c. queue.

    b. periwig.
    d. toupee. _____

132. The best form of advertising for your barbershop or services are:

    a. giveaway promotional items.
    c. social media posts.

    b. satisfied clients.
    d. television ads. _____

133. To chemically oxidize hair, thio relaxing products require a(n):

    a. texturizer.
    c. neutralizer.

    b. activator.
    d. moisturizer. _____

134. The wrapping pattern where all rods within a panel are positioned in the same direction on equal-size bases is the:
a. curvature wrap.
c. basic wrap.
b. piggyback wrap.
d. bricklay wrap.
_____

135. The pigment that lies under the natural hair color is:
a. artificial pigment.
c. foundation pigment.
b. contributing pigment.
d. natural pigment.
_____

136. Replacement hair that can last a lifetime if the service is performed properly is:
a. cell regenerated.
c. synthetic.
b. transplanted.
d. cover-up.
_____

137. The night before an examination you should avoid:
a. rest.
c. reading notes.
b. test-taking strategies.
d. cramming.
_____

138. Hydroxide relaxers can have a pH over:
a. 13.0.
c. 10.0.
b. 9.6.
d. 9.0.
_____

139. The technique that increases the size of the curl as it nears the scalp area, with a tighter curl at the ends, is:
a. croquignole perm wrapping.
c. spiral wrapping.
b. double-end wrapping.
d. bookend wrapping.
_____

140. Colors created by mixing equal amounts of two primary colors are:
a. quaternary.
c. tertiary.
b. secondary.
d. complementary.
_____

141. An oral medication for hair replacement, with potential side effects of weight gain and loss of sexual function, is:
a. finasteride.
c. Rogaine.
b. loniten.
d. minoxidil.
_____

142. The average time a potential employer will spend scanning your resume is:
a. 45 seconds.
c. 20 seconds.
b. 1 minute.
d. 5 minutes.
_____

143. When waving lotions/solutions break disulfide bonds, it is called:
a. lanthionization.
c. reduction.
b. oxidation.
d. reformation.
_____

144. Waves that require an outside heat source to activate chemical reactions and processing are:
- **a.** exothermic.
- **b.** cold.
- **c.** acid-balanced.
- **d.** endothermic.   ____

145. A nonoxidizing haircolor that washes out or fades within a few weeks is considered:
- **a.** temporary.
- **b.** demipermanent.
- **c.** permanent.
- **d.** semipermanent.   ____

146. A service that could be offered in the barbershop is:
- **a.** scalp reduction.
- **b.** hair transplantation.
- **c.** flap surgery.
- **d.** low-light laser therapy.   ____

147. Skills mastered at other jobs that can be put to use in a new position are:
- **a.** transferable skills.
- **b.** academic skills.
- **c.** test-taking skills.
- **d.** career skills.   ____

148. Chemical texture products that break chemical bonds and soften and expand the hair are:
- **a.** acidic substances.
- **b.** alkaline substances.
- **c.** alkanolamines.
- **d.** mercaptamines.   ____

149. A limp or weak wave formation with undefined ridges within the S pattern results from:
- **a.** overprocessing.
- **b.** underprocessing.
- **c.** reconditioning.
- **d.** faster processing.   ____

150. Hair that absorbs the base color of the toner is:
- **a.** overlightened.
- **b.** gray.
- **c.** underlightened.
- **d.** pre-lightened.   ____

Chapter 1 THE HISTORY OF BARBERING

1. a	pg.06	LO1	8. a	pg.12	LO2	15. c	pg.15	LO3
2. c	pg.07	LO1	9. b	pg.12	LO2	16. b	pg.16	LO4
3. d	pg.08	LO1	10. b	pg.12	LO2	17. a	pg.16	LO4
4. a	pg.09	LO1	11. d	pg.14	LO3	18. d	pg.17	LO4
5. b	pg.10	LO1	12. c	pg.15	LO3	19. a	pg.16	LO4
6. b	pg.11	LO2	13. a	pg.15	LO3	20. d	pg.17	LO4
7. c	pg.11	LO2	14. a	pg.15	LO3			

Chapter 2 LIFE SKILLS

1. a	pg.24	LO1	8. a	pg.28	LO4	15. d	pg.35	LO7
2. a	pg.24	LO1	9. d	pg.30	LO5	16. b	pg.35	LO7
3. c	pg.26	LO2	10. b	pg.31	LO5	17. a	pg.36	LO7
4. c	pg.25	LO2	11. d	pg.31	LO5	18. c	pg.36	LO8
5. b	pg.27	LO3	12. a	pg.32	LO6	19. d	pg.36	LO8
6. a	pg.27	LO3	13. b	pg.34	LO6			
7. c	pg.29	LO4	14. c	pg.32	LO6			

Chapter 3 PROFESSIONAL IMAGE

1. c	pg.42	LO1	13. d	pg.45	LO3	25. b	pg.50	LO4
2. a	pg.42	LO1	14. b	pg.45	LO3	26. b	pg.49	LO4
3. c	pg.41	LO1	15. d	pg.46	LO3	27. d	pg.47	LO4
4. b	pg.41	LO1	16. a	pg.46	LO3	28. c	pg.49	LO4
5. b	pg.41	LO1	17. b	pg.45	LO3	29. a	pg.47	LO4
6. b	pg.42	LO2	18. c	pg.44	LO3	30. b	pg.48	LO4
7. d	pg.43	LO2	19. a	pg.45	LO3	31. c	pg.47	LO4
8. c	pg.42	LO2	20. b	pg.45	LO3	32. d	pg.48	LO4
9. a	pg.42	LO2	21. d	pg.45	LO3	33. b	pg.48	LO4
10. c	pg.43	LO2	22. c	pg.46	LO3	34. c	pg.50	LO4
11. a	pg.44	LO3	23. b	pg.48	LO4	35. a	pg.50	LO4
12. c	pg.45	LO3	24. a	pg.48	LO4	36. c	pg.48	LO4

Chapter 4 INFECTION CONTROL: PRINCPLES AND PRACTICES

1. b	pg.57	LO1	9. c	pg.58	LO1	17. c	pg.63	LO2
2. c	pg.59	LO1	10. d	pg.60	LO1	18. b	pg.66	LO2
3. a	pg.58	LO1	11. a	pg.63	LO2	19. a	pg.66	LO2
4. d	pg.62	LO1	12. b	pg.64	LO2	20. c	pg.63	LO2
5. c	pg.62	LO1	13. c	pg.65	LO2	21. b	pg.67	LO2
6. d	pg.60	LO1	14. b	pg.65	LO2	22. d	pg.67	LO2
7. b	pg.62	LO1	15. a	pg.65	LO2	23. c	pg.67	LO2
8. a	pg.60	LO1	16. d	pg.63	LO2	24. a	pg.66	LO2

Chapter 5   IMPLEMENTS, TOOLS, AND EQUIPMENT

Chapter 6 GENERAL ANATOMY AND PHYSIOLOGY

1. b	pg.144	LO1	23. a	pg.152	LO5	45. a	pg.158	LO5
2. d	pg.144	LO1	24. d	pg.152	LO5	46. b	pg.159	LO5
3. c	pg.145	LO1	25. c	pg.154	LO5	47. c	pg.167	LO5
4. d	pg.145	LO2	26. b	pg.154	LO5	48. d	pg.166	LO:
5. a	pg.145	LO2	27. a	pg.155	LO:	49. a	pg.165	LO5
6. c	pg.146	LO2	28. d	pg.156	LO5	50. b	pg.157	LO5
7. b	pg.145	LO2	29. c	pg.156	LO5	51. c	pg.158	LO5
8. d	pg.147	LO3	30. b	pg.151	LO5	52. d	pg.165	LO5
9. c	pg.147	LO3	31. a	pg.149	LO5	53. c	pg.149	LO5
10. b	pg.147	LO3	32. d	pg.150	LO5	54. a	pg.151	LO5
11. d	pg.147	LO3	33. c	pg.165	LO5	55. b	pg.151	LO5
12. b	pg.147	LO3	34. a	pg.167	LO5	56. c	pg.165	LO5
13. c	pg.147	LO4	35. b	pg.161	LO5	57. d	pg.164	LO5
14. c	pg.147	LO4	36. c	pg.166	LO5	58. b	pg.162	LO5
15. a	pg.148	LO5	37. a	pg.165	LO5	59. a	pg.161	LO5
16. c	pg.149	LO5	38. d	pg.165	LO5	60. b	pg.161	LO5
17. b	pg.150	LO5	39. b	pg.160	LO5	61. d	pg.160	LO5
18. d	pg.149	LO5	40. a	pg.161	LO5	62. c	pg.158	LO5
19. a	pg.151	LO5	41. c	pg.162	LO5	63. b	pg.151	LO5
20. c	pg.151	LO5	42. a	pg.157	LO5	64. d	pg.150	LO5
21. d	pg.151	LO5	43. c	pg.157	LO5	65. b	pg.158	LO5
22. b	pg.150	LO5	44. d	pg.157	LO5			

Chapter 7 BASICS OF CHEMISTRY

1. c	pg.179	LO1	17. d	pg.182	LO4	33. b	pg.188	LO6
2. a	pg.179	LO1	18. a	pg.182	LO4	34. d	pg.188	LO7
3. b	pg.179	LO1	19. c	pg.182	LO4	35. b	pg.189	LO7
4. d	pg.179	LO1	20. a	pg.183	LO4	36. c	pg.190	LO7
5. c	pg.179	LO2	21. b	pg.183	LO3	37. c	pg.192	LO8
6. b	pg.179	LO2	22. d	pg.184	LO3	38. a	pg.193	LO8
7. d	pg.180	LO2	23. b	pg.184	LO3	39. b	pg.193	LO8
8. a	pg.181	LO2	24. c	pg.185	LO5	40. c	pg.194	LO9
9. d	pg.180	LO2	25. a	pg.186	LO5	41. d	pg.195	LO9
10. c	pg.180	LO2	26. d	pg.187	LO5	42. b	pg.196	LO10
11. a	pg.181	LO3	27. b	pg.186	LO5	43. a	pg.195	LO10
12. c	pg.181	LO3	28. a	pg.185	LO5	44. c	pg.198	LO10
13. b	pg.181	LO3	29. c	pg.188	LO6	45. a	pg.199	LO10
14. d	pg.182	LO3	30. d	pg.188	LO6	46. d	pg.199	LO10
15. c	pg.182	LO3	31. c	pg.188	LO6	47. c	pg.197	LO10
16. b	pg.182	LO4	32. a	pg.188	LO6	48. b	pg.198	LO10

Chapter 8 BASICS OF ELECTRICITY

1. b	pg.206	LO:NA	11. a	pg.209	LO3	21. a	pg.214	LO5	
2. c	pg.207	LO2	12. d	pg.209	LO3	22. c	pg.215	LO5	
3. a	pg.206	LO1	13. c	pg.211	LO3	23. a	pg.214	LO5	
4. d	pg.206	LO1	14. d	pg.211	LO3	24. b	pg.214	LO5	
5. b	pg.206	LO1	15. b	pg.211	LO4	25. d	pg.215	LO5	
6. c	pg.208	LO2	16. d	pg.212	LO4	26. c	pg.216	LO6	
7. d	pg.207	LO2	17. a	pg.212	LO4	27. a	pg.217	LO6	
8. a	pg.208	LO2	18. c	pg.212	LO4	28. b	pg.217	LO6	
9. b	pg.209	LO2	19. d	pg.213	LO4	29. d	pg.216	LO6	
10. c	pg.209	LO3	20. c	pg.213	LO4	30. c	pg.217	LO6	

Chapter 9 THE SKIN – STRUCTURES, DISORDERS, AND DISEASES

1. b	pg.222	LO1	24. c	pg.233	LO3	46. d	pg.238	LO7
2. c	pg.223	LO1	25. d	pg.232	LO3	47. b	pg.239	LO7
3. d	pg.223	LO1	26. b	pg.233	LO3	48. a	pg.239	LO7
4. a	pg.224	LO1	27. a	pg.230	LO3	49. c	pg.238	LO7
5. c	pg.225	LO1	28. b	pg.233	LO3	50. b	pg.239	LO7
6. d	pg.228	LO1	29. c	pg.236,	LO4	51. a	pg.239	LO8
7. c	pg.225	LO1		237		52. c	pg.239	LO8
8. a	pg.225	LO1	30. a	pg.236	LO4	53. d	pg.240	LO8
9. b	pg.225	LO1	31. b	pg.237	LO4	54. b	pg.240	LO:NA
10. a	pg.226	LO1	32. d	pg.236	LO4	55. c	pg.240	LO:NA
11. c	pg.226	LO1	33. c	pg.236	LO4	56. b	pg.240	LO8
12. d	pg.226	LO1	34. d	pg.235	LO5	57. a	pg.239	LO8
13. b	pg.227	LO1	35. b	pg.234	LO5	58. d	pg.239	LO8
14. a	pg.228	LO2	36. a	pg.236	LO5	59. a	pg.239	LO8
15. d	pg.229	LO2	37. c	pg.236	LO5	60. b	pg.240	LO:NA
16. c	pg.229	LO2	38. d	pg.236	LO5	61. c	pg.240	LO:NA
17. b	pg.229	LO2	39. b	pg.238	LO6	62. a	pg.238	LO7
18. c	pg.228	LO2	40. a	pg.238	LO6	63. d	pg.238	LO6
19. d	pg.232	LO3	41. c	pg.238	LO6	64. b	pg.238	LO6
20. a	pg.230	LO3	42. d	pg.238	LO6	65. a	pg.237	LO8
21. b	pg.230	LO3	43. a	pg.238	LO6	66. c	pg.237	LO8
22. c	pg.232	LO3	44. b	pg.238	LO6			
23. a	pg.231	LO3	45. c	pg.238	LO7			

Chapter 10 PROPERTIES AND DISORDERS OF THE HAIR AND SCALP

1. b	pg.248	LO1	6. c	pg.249	LO2	12. d	pg.250	LO3
2. a	pg.249	LO1	7. b	pg.250	LO2	13. a	pg.251	LO3
3. a	pg.249	LO1	8. a	pg.250	LO2	14. c	pg.252	LO3
4. c	pg.249	LO1	9. d	pg.250	LO2	15. a	pg.252	LO3
5. d	pg.248,	LO1	10. b	pg.250	LO2	16. c	pg.252	LO3
	249		11. c	pg.250	LO3	17. d	pg.253	LO3

Chapter 11   TREATMENT OF THE HAIR AND SCALP

Chapter 12   MEN'S FACIAL MASSAGE AND TREATMENTS

42. b	pg.318	LO8	54. b	pg.318	LO8	66. b	pg.321	LO9
43. a	pg.317	LO8	55. c	pg.318	LO8	67. a	pg.321	LO9
44. d	pg.317	LO8	56. d	pg.320	LO9	68. d	pg.322	LO9
45. c	pg.314	LO8	57. c	pg.321	LO9	69. c	pg.322	LO9
46. b	pg.317	LO8	58. b	pg.322	LO9	70. c	pg.323	LO9
47. a	pg.317	LO8	59. a	pg.322	LO9	71. b	pg.323	LO9
48. d	pg.315	LO8	60. d	pg.325	LO9	72. a	pg.323	LO9
49. c	pg.315	LO8	61. c	pg.325	LO9	73. c	pg.325	LO9
50. c	pg.318	LO8	62. d	pg.323	LO9	74. d	pg.320	LO9
51. c	pg.316	LO8	63. b	pg.323	LO9	75. a	pg.320	LO9
52. d	pg.314	LO8	64. a	pg.322	LO9	76. c	pg.325	LO9
53. a	pg.318	LO8	65. c	pg.322	LO9			

Chapter 13   SHAVING AND FACIAL-HAIR DESIGN

1. b	pg.339	LO1	16. b	pg.345	LO3	32. c	pg.348	LO3
2. c	pg.338, 339	LO1	17. d	pg.348	LO3	33. d	pg.348	LO3
			18. c	pg.348	LO3	34. a	pg.348	LO3
3. a	pg.339	LO1	19. a	pg.349	LO3	35. c	pg.349	LO3
4. d	pg.340	LO1	20. d	pg.349	LO3	36. b	pg.349	LO3
5. c	pg.339	LO1	21. b	pg.350	LO4	37. d	pg.351	LO4
6. b	pg.339	LO1	22. c	pg.351	LO4	38. c	pg.349	LO3
7. a	pg.339	LO1	23. b	pg.343	LO3	39. b	pg.348	LO3
8. d	pg.339	LO1	24. a	pg.342	LO3	40. a	pg.348	LO3
9. c	pg.339	LO1	25. c	pg.343	LO3	41. c	pg.352	LO5
10. b	pg.340	LO1	26. d	pg.370	LO3	42. b	pg.352	LO5
11. c	pg.340	LO2	27. a	pg.347	LO3	43. d	pg.352	LO5
12. d	pg.340	LO2	28. c	pg.352	LO5	44. c	pg.352	LO5
13. a	pg.340	LO2	29. b	pg.342	LO3	45. b	pg.352	LO5
14. b	pg.342	LO2	30. a	pg.343	LO3	46. a	pg.352	LO5
15. c	pg.342	LO2	31. b	pg.347	LO3			

Chapter 14   MEN'S HAIRCUTTING AND STYLING

1. b	pg.385	LO1	11. c	pg.391	LO2	21. b	pg.397	LO5
2. d	pg.385	LO1	12. d	pg.388	LO2	22. d	pg.395	LO5
3. c	pg.386	LO1	13. a	pg.388	LO2	23. a	pg.396	LO5
4. a	pg.388	LO2	14. b	pg.393	LO3	24. c	pg.396	LO5
5. c	pg.389	LO2	15. a	pg.393	LO3	25. d	pg.395	LO5
6. b	pg.389	LO2	16. b	pg.393	LO3	26. a	pg.397	LO6
7. d	pg.388	LO2	17. d	pg.394	LO4	27. b	pg.398	LO6
8. a	pg.390	LO2	18. c	pg.393	LO4	28. c	pg.398	LO6
9. c	pg.390	LO2	19. a	pg.394	LO4	29. d	pg.400	LO6
10. d	pg.390	LO2	20. c	pg.395	LO5	30. a	pg.400	LO6

Chapter 15   MEN'S HAIR REPLACEMENT

Chapter 16   WOMEN'S HAIRCUTTING AND STYLING

Chapter 17 CHEMICAL TEXTURE SERVICES

1. b	pg.579	LO1	24. b	pg.589	LO6	48. a	pg.596	LO7
2. c	pg.579	LO1	25. a	pg.592	LO6	49. a	pg.597	LO7
3. d	pg.578,	LO1	26. c	pg.589	LO6	50. b	pg.598	LO7
	579		27. d	pg.589	LO6	51. c	pg.606	LO8
4. a	pg.580	LO2	28. b	pg.589	LO6	52. d	pg.606	LO8
5. a	pg.580	LO2	29. b	pg.589	LO6	53. b	pg.606	LO8
6. a	pg.579	LO2	30. a	pg.589	LO6	54. a	pg.607	LO9
7. d	pg.582	LO3	31. c	pg.593	LO7	55. d	pg.606	LO9
8. b	pg.583	LO3	32. b	pg.593	LO7	56. b	pg.607	LO10
9. c	pg.583	LO3	33. b	pg.593	LO7	57. c	pg.608	LO10
10. a	pg.583	LO3	34. a	pg.594	LO7	58. d	pg.609	LO11
11. d	pg.582	LO3	35. c	pg.594	LO7	59. a	pg.609	LO11
12. b	pg.585	LO4	36. d	pg.594	LO7	60. c	pg.609	LO11
13. c	pg.587	LO5	37. b	pg.595	LO7	61. b	pg.609	LO11
14. d	pg.587	LO5	38. a	pg.595	LO7	62. d	pg.609	LO11
15. c	pg.587	LO5	39. c	pg.595	LO7	63. b	pg.610	LO12
16. b	pg.586	LO4	40. d	pg.595	LO7	64. a	pg.610	LO12
17. d	pg.587	LO5	41. c	pg.592	LO7	65. c	pg.611	LO12
18. a	pg.585	LO5	42. d	pg.595	LO7	66. d	pg.610	LO12
19. d	pg.585	LO5	43. b	pg.593	LO7	67. d	pg.610	LO12
20. b	pg.586	LO5	44. a	pg.594	LO7	68. b	pg.610	LO12
21. c	pg.588	LO6	45. c	pg.596	LO7	69. d	pg.610	LO12
22. a	pg.589	LO6	46. d	pg.596	LO7	70. c	pg.611	LO12
23. d	pg.588	LO6	47. b	pg.600	LO7			

Chapter 18 HAIRCOLORING AND LIGHTENING

1. a	pg.643	LO1	16. c	pg.647	LO2	31. d	pg.658	LO4
2. c	pg.643	LO1	17. d	pg.646	LO2	32. a	pg.660	LO4
3. d	pg.644	LO1	18. a	pg.647	LO2	33. b	pg.660	LO4
4. b	pg.644	LO1	19. d	pg.646	LO2	34. c	pg.659	LO4
5. b	pg.643	LO1	20. d	pg.649	LO3	35. a	pg.658	LO4
6. c	pg.643	LO1	21. b	pg.649	LO3	36. b	pg.661	LO4
7. d	pg.644	LO1	22. a	pg.652	LO3	37. d	pg.662	LO5
8. a	pg.643	LO1	23. a	pg.655	LO3	38. c	pg.663	LO5
9. c	pg.643	LO1	24. c	pg.654	LO3	39. d	pg.666	LO5
10. b	pg.644	LO1	25. b	pg.654	LO3	40. c	pg.662	LO5
11. c	pg.645	LO2	26. d	pg.654	LO3	41. d	pg.662	LO5
12. d	pg.645	LO2	27. a	pg.656	LO3	42. b	pg.662	LO5
13. a	pg.645	LO2	28. c	pg.655	LO3	43. a	pg.663	LO5
14. b	pg.645	LO2	29. d	pg.653	LO4	44. c	pg.662	LO5
15. b	pg.646	LO2	30. c	pg.657	LO4	45. d	pg.667	LO6

Chapter 19 PREPARING FOR LICENSURE AND EMPLOYMENT

Chapter 20 WORKING BEHIND THE CHAIR

Chapter 21 THE BUSINESS OF BARBERING

SAMPLE STATE BOARD EXAMINATION TEST 1

1. a	31. b	61. b	91. b	121. c
2. b	32. d	62. c	92. b	122. a
3. b	33. c	63. a	93. b	123. d
4. d	34. c	64. d	94. d	124. a
5. d	35. a	65. c	95. b	125. b
6. a	36. a	66. d	96. a	126. a
7. d	37. a	67. b	97. c	127. c
8. b	38. b	68. d	98. a	128. b
9. a	39. a	69. d	99. a	129. a
10. d	40. b	70. d	100. b	130. c
11. b	41. b	71. b	101. b	131. d
12. a	42. b	72. d	102. c	132. c
13. a	43. a	73. b	103. c	133. c
14. b	44. d	74. b	104. a	134. c
15. c	45. c	75. d	105. c	135. b
16. a	46. a	76. b	106. c	136. a
17. d	47. a	77. a	107. b	137. d
18. b	48. c	78. c	108. c	138. b
19. b	49. a	79. c	109. d	139. b
20. a	50. c	80. c	110. c	140. d
21. b	51. d	81. a	111. c	141. d
22. c	52. a	82. d	112. a	142. a
23. a	53. c	83. a	113. c	143. d
24. d	54. a	84. c	114. c	144. c
25. c	55. c	85. c	115. c	145. d
26. b	56. a	86. b	116. d	146. d
27. b	57. d	87. c	117. b	147. b
28. d	58. c	88. d	118. d	148. c
29. b	59. d	89. c	119. a	149. a
30. d	60. b	90. c	120. b	150. d

SAMPLE STATE BOARD EXAMINATION TEST 2

1. c	31. c	61. b	91. c	121. b
2. a	32. b	62. d	92. a	122. a
3. b	33. c	63. d	93. a	123. d
4. c	34. b	64. b	94. c	124. b
5. d	35. a	65. a	95. b	125. a
6. a	36. a	66. d	96. d	126. b
7. c	37. c	67. d	97. b	127. c
8. d	38. d	68. c	98. a	128. c
9. d	39. d	69. b	99. b	129. c
10. d	40. a	70. d	100. b	130. a
11. d	41. b	71. d	101. a	131. c
12. b	42. c	72. a	102. a	132. c
13. c	43. a	73. d	103. c	133. b
14. d	44. a	74. b	104. a	134. a
15. b	45. a	75. b	105. b	135. d
16. d	46. c	76. b	106. a	136. d
17. d	47. c	77. d	107. d	137. d
18. d	48. c	78. b	108. c	138. c
19. c	49. d	79. b	109. a	139. d
20. d	50. a	80. a	110. d	140. c
21. a	51. b	81. a	111. c	141. c
22. d	52. b	82. a	112. a	142. b
23. b	53. c	83. d	113. c	143. d
24. b	54. b	84. a	114. b	144. b
25. a	55. c	85. b	115. d	145. a
26. b	56. d	86. c	116. d	146. a
27. b	57. a	87. d	117. c	147. b
28. c	58. a	88. a	118. a	148. c
29. d	59. c	89. b	119. d	149. c
30. a	60. c	90. c	120. a	150. c

1. a	31. b	61. c	91. b	121. b
2. b	32. c	62. d	92. c	122. b
3. b	33. a	63. d	93. b	123. d
4. a	34. b	64. c	94. b	124. b
5. d	35. b	65. c	95. c	125. a
6. a	36. b	66. d	96. c	126. b
7. a	37. c	67. b	97. a	127. b
8. c	38. d	68. c	98. a	128. a
9. d	39. b	69. c	99. b	129. b
10. d	40. a	70. a	100. a	130. a
11. b	41. d	71. a	101. b	131. d
12. b	42. d	72. b	102. b	132. b
13. d	43. d	73. b	103. b	133. c
14. d	44. b	74. b	104. a	134. c
15. c	45. d	75. a	105. a	135. b
16. c	46. b	76. c	106. b	136. b
17. a	47. a	77. c	107. c	137. d
18. c	48. c	78. d	108. a	138. a
19. d	49. d	79. b	109. b	139. a
20. b	50. c	80. b	110. b	140. b
21. a	51. b	81. c	111. b	141. a
22. d	52. c	82. b	112. c	142. c
23. c	53. d	83. c	113. c	143. c
24. a	54. d	84. b	114. c	144. d
25. d	55. d	85. a	115. d	145. d
26. b	56. a	86. c	116. c	146. d
27. c	57. c	87. c	117. c	147. a
28. c	58. c	88. d	118. c	148. b
29. d	59. a	89. d	119. d	149. b
30. c	60. b	90. d	120. b	150. a